The Natural Way
to
Better Eyesight

THE NATURAL WAY
TO
BETTER EYESIGHT

by

J. I. Rodale

RODALE PRESS, INC. EMMAUS, PA. 18049

Table of Contents

Introduction

I AM NOT a believer in introductions, forewords, or prefaces. They are a wall between the reader and the book, not to mention the author. An author who writes involved, wordy introductions is doing himself and his cause a great injustice, while antagonizing his reader at the very point when he needs his confidence. It is like putting on your overcoat to keep cool.

What an author has to say belongs in the book, because if he is going to waste his ammunition in the foreword he will have that much less to say when he has to say it later on, or suffer the sin of repetition. There is many an introduction which really is chapter one, so why not call it that and be done with it?

The trouble is that no scientific research has ever been done to improve or find a substitute for introductions. Our best brains are wasted in planning to go to the moon and in figuring out splashdowns. Scientists will spend years figuring out the sense of rotation which exists in a cyclone or whether the two deflective forces involved are additive, or whatever; but they will read long introductions without complaining to their subconscious about it and without starting a project to improve the situation. Aristotle's introductions are still the vogue today.

Then there are books with whole series of introductions. I have one before me which contains 86 pages of meat and 124 pages of prefaces. There is the preface to the Dover edition, the publisher's comment, prefaces to the first, second, and third editions, and one by Lady Eastlake. If this continues, I will begin reading my books in Japanese fashion, starting from the end and working my way forward, page by page, to the point of no return—the foreword.

But in spite of all this the average reader, strange creature, still wants his introduction. He feels that it is part of the anatomy of the book, like the binding or the dust jacket. He is guilty of a complacent conformity, not realizing that the world is changing.

So, if I wish to sell books I will have to conform; but in my conformity I will give the world introductions that will be unforgettable. They will be more like a warm-up, as they say in psychodrama. No filler for me. I will begin as an after-dinner speaker. Here goes:

On the way to writing this book I met two burglars on a street corner, who were talking to each other, and one was saying:

"I need eyeglasses."

"What makes you think so?" asked the second burglar.

"Well, I was twirling the knob of a safe when suddenly a dance orchestra began to play."

So, after you have stopped laughing, you may turn to Chapter 1, which is about sunflower-seed eating as an aid to the tissues of the eyes. Many newspaper writers have been jokingly irreverent on the subject, cautioning their readers not to eat too many of these seeds lest they might suddenly find themselves chirping like birds. The joke shows what a poor sense of humor they have—the writers, not the birds, with apologies to Aristophanes.

I think this introduction has gone far enough, so turn the page and begin reading.

J. I. RODALE

Chapter 1

Sunflower Seeds
and the Eyes

ONCE I EXPERIMENTED with chickens on my farm, dividing them into two groups which were fed a uniform diet, except that one group received sunflower seeds, but the other did not. The feathers of these birds became more shiny and colorful, which is a sign of better health. I decided to eat sunflower seeds, too, to see what they would do for me. In about a week, I noticed a very startling thing. A slight, intermittent quiver in my left eye went away. I usually suffered from this only in the winter, when there is little opportunity for exercise or to be in the sun. This condition has never returned.

My eyes are not my strongest point. In the winter I used to have trouble in walking on snow-blanketed roads. Before I became aware of the value of eating sunflower seeds, I left the house on the farm one day for a walk, but had to return after being out only a moment because the great brightness of the snow interfered with my vision. In fact, it made the snow seem a pink color. After being on the sunflower diet for about a month, I noticed I could walk in the snow without distress. A little while later my car broke down and I had to walk over a mile on a snow-covered highway in bright sunshine. I had no trouble at all for the first three-quarters of the way. On the last stretch, my eyes smarted a little.

Because of my new ability to stand snow glare, I imagined that sunflower seeds must be rich in vitamin A; but when I checked, I discovered that they contained only small amounts of this vitamin but were unusually rich in vitamin B. And it is for this reason that they give the eyes a "resistance to light." Quoting from a French medical journal, "It seems that riboflavin [which is vitamin B_2] protects the cones in the eye from excess light, and that is the reason why it is found in the pigmented cells of the retina. It is probable that the pigment plays a very important role here. A deficiency in riboflavin brings about a lessening of visual acuity."

In pellagra, it is an injury to the cones of the eye which makes them hypersensitive to light. During World War II, there was a condition of "camp eyes" and sun blindness which afflicted prisoners in concentration camps, and it was always traced to a pellagra condition caused by vitamin B deficiencies in the diet.

Hulled sunflower seeds are now available from many sources, so there is no need to bother with shelling the seeds. If you are engaged in activities out

12

in the sunshine, such as working, playing tennis, yachting, frequenting beaches, etc., start eating these seeds—a small handful or two a day—and see if you won't be able to discard your sunglasses. You will be convinced that there is something in sunflower seeds that will enable you to withstand the glare of a tropical sun without using sunglasses.

As my own personal opinion, and not to be taken scientifically, I will hazard a guess that it is something in addition to the vitamin B that exerts this mysterious power over the eyes. There is a phenomenon called heliotropism that can be observed in the sunflower. As soon as the head of the sunflower is formed, it always faces the sun. As the sun swings its orbit across the heavens, the sunflower head turns with it, until, late in the day, it is facing due west to absorb the last few rays of the dying sun. The seed, therefore, is just drenched with sun vitality.

A friend has an electric machine that tests the electric potential of plants. He has found that foods growing in the sun contain a higher electric potential than foods (like the potato) that grow in the ground. He also has found that apples growing on the outside of the tree, in the sun, have much more electric potential than those growing in the interior of the tree where it is shady.

I cannot talk about sunflower seeds without talking about Russia. Ivan does not know their nutritional advantages, but he has always eaten them with zest. Children in Russia prefer sunflower seeds to candy.

There are many reasons why the sunflower seed is

13

a valuable food and should be included in everyone's diet. In the first place, nature protects it with a casing. It therefore stores well and loses very little vitamin value over long periods. When you remove the outer shell, you have a concentrated bit of healthy nourishment. It tastes almost as delicious a year after harvesting as on the day it was cut down. I have eaten with relish raw wheat seed on harvest day, but a month later it had already lost some of its palatability.

Second, you eat the sunflower seed raw. It comes to you in virgin form. Nutritionists all agree that cooking, however skillfully done, destroys some of the vitamins.

This plant is one of the easiest to grow. You have never heard of anyone spraying poisons on it because it is very hardy and is highly resistant to disease.

The American Indian found wide use for the seed of the sunflower, which he employed as food, hair oil, and soap. Members of the Lewis and Clark expedition found much evidence of this. In their journal for July 17, 1805, when they were in Montana, there is recorded the following:

"Along the bottoms, which have a covering of high grass, we observe the *sunflower* blooming in great abundance. The Indians of the Missouri, more especially those who do not cultivate maize, make great use of the seed of this plant for bread, or in thickening their soup. They first parch and then pound it between two stones, until it is reduced to a fine meal. Sometimes they add a portion of water, and drink it thus diluted; at other times they add a sufficient pro-

14

portion of marrow-grease to reduce it to the consistency of common dough, and eat it in that manner. This last composition we preferred to all the rest, and thought it at the time a very palatable dish."

Note the use of marrow-grease, a product made from bones.

Columbus had long before noted how popular the sunflower was with the Indians and he was instrumental in introducing it into Europe. Today, though this seed is very popular in many parts of Europe, it is practically unknown in this country as a food for human beings.

I will eat a handful of sunflower seeds every day for the rest of my life, and I advise you do likewise. And if you have the tiniest bit of grass, you ought to grow your own sunflower plants organically. If you don't have any compost, use a liberal amount of dried blood and bone meal, which are available at chain stores, nurseries, and seed stores. Even with compost, add a liberal amount of dried blood and bone meal. If you can get some kind of seaweed fertilizer, or rotted manure, so much the better.

Chapter 2

Those Fabulous Sunflower-seed-eating Russians

You CANNOT TALK to any Russian about sunflower seeds without his going into ecstatic raptures on the subject. Eating what we used to call Polly Seeds is a national pastime there, indulged by young and old, high and low. The rank and file in Russia do not seem to know that it is possessed of inestimable nutritional advantages, but they eat it with zest. I know of no American food that is eaten so regularly—not even candy. The Russians are big and broad-boned, and their teeth on the average are in much better shape than ours in this country. Their general intelligence compares favorably with the rest of the nations of the world.

On holidays Russians walk the streets and promenade in the parks with their pockets bulging with sunflower seeds. A friend of mine who came from Russia many years ago tells me that the last recollection he has of his country was a hillside on which a group of young folks were lounging and munching sunflower seeds. He can still see their enchanting silhouette against the skyline and hear the crackling of the seeds. That means Russia to him.

In Russia the sunflower is big business (as it is also rapidly becoming in Argentina). There are many factories there for extracting oil from these seeds and for making potash from the stalks. There are also processing plants that use the residues for making animal feeds. Russian table oil is practically 100 per cent obtained from sunflower seeds, and it is said to be of superior quality because it does not solidify very easily.

In the old Czarist days in Russia, every soldier in the field received what was known as iron rations. It consisted of a bag of sunflower seeds weighing 1 kilogram (about 2 1/5 pounds). Soldiers sometimes lived exclusively on these seeds. The army evidently was aware that they contained important nutritional values.

One reader (Elton R. Graybiel of Los Angeles, Calif.) who saw this fact in an old article of mine wrote me on April 5, 1945:

"I have checked the iron requirements in sunflower seeds and 2 lbs. contains .021 grams of iron, which equals 21 milligrams, the daily requirement of iron for a man, and for a woman of the same weight in adult life she requires 15 mgs. of iron daily.

"My attention was directed to this fact by a comment in our *Organic Gardening* about the former Czar of Russia giving to the soldiers 2 lbs. of sun-

17

flower seeds daily in their ration, so I checked it at once and find it an ample source of iron."

It is established etiquette in Russia that these seeds may be eaten everywhere and under almost any conditions. Every home has a bowlful prominently placed. A Russian recently described for me the recognized etiquette for handling the seeds. In a home you place the shells in a neat pile on the table where you are eating them. On the street you may munch them as you walk, your pockets bulging with them. You accumulate the shells in the left hand, and when you have enough, you throw them into some obscure corner. I suppose it must represent a tremendous street-cleaning problem. In contrast to this, I came across an extremely amusing item in a newspaper feature called "It's the Law," by Dick Hyman, which stated, "The eating of sunflower seeds on the streets of Endicott, Washington, or in its business houses is prohibited."

Dr. Ehrenfried Pfeiffer writes me, "The South-Russians, Turks, Arabs, etc. about the Black Sea and Asia Minor are always chewing sunflower and cucumber seeds, as we do gum (as I witnessed myself, slipping on spittings of them everywhere over there), and ascribe their splendid health to it, who knows why?"

I have often wondered what the effect of this is on the Russian eyesight, and I obtained my answer when I recently saw a moving picture called *Inside Russia.* Rarely was a person to be seen who wore glasses. From what I observed, I would say that less than 10 per cent of the Russians wear glasses. In our country, 60 per cent of all adults are doomed to wear them, and the tendency is increasing. In the event of war between the United States and Russia, does this fact have some significance?

Chapter 3

Sunflower Seed Correspondence with Readers

IN THE APRIL, 1944, issue of *Organic Gardening* magazine I published the details of my experiences with sunflower seeds. The reaction of my readers was immediate and electric. The article was reprinted by three health publications. It was also reprinted in England by the *News Letter on Compost.* Letters poured in by the hundreds. Many stated they were going to grow sunflowers for food. Thousands started to eat these seeds. The correspondence has been both enjoyable and satisfying. Here are a few representative letters:

October 28, 1944

Dear Mr. Rodale:

You asked that I note any difference in flavor in the organically raised sunflower seeds and my answer is decidedly in the affirmative. They are free from the slight bitterness that all the seeds I have purchased in both the seed stores and from a farmer in the market, have had. In addition the flavor itself is fuller and more pleasing. Fortunately, I had a few of our own on hand and had just purchased a pound in the market, so my sister and I had an excellent opportunity to make comparisons. We felt like the "tea tasters" of which we have read.

Incidentally, would you care to add to your collection of sunflower seed cures? My sister had had a chronic and most stubborn "gum boil" (or whatever is the correct name of those annoying gum sores) and it had been with her for many months when we started eating sunflower seeds. That was about 10 months ago. We each eat a good sized handful each day and after a month or two the gum sore disappeared and there has been no recurrence.

Lora K. Alessandroni
Philadelphia, Pa.

January 3, 1945

Dear Mr. Rodale:

My own experience with sunflower seeds has been interesting if not conclusive. As I recall, I visit my dentist once each year and he finds one or two small cavities. At my last visit, a month or so ago, he found no cavities after not seeing me for thirteen and one half months. For the last ten of these thirteen and one half months, I have been eating about two heaping tablespoons full of commercially grown sunflower seeds each day.

> Dr. Juan Amon
> Wilkins Natural School
> Isle of Pines, Cuba

October 15, 1944

Dear Mr. Rodale:

I have been eating sunflower seeds for several months and while my difficulty is an organic one—yet I have noticed one thing—that tired feeling I always carried around with me—plus the soreness in muscles have diminished to a very marked degree.

> B. H. Toenjes
> St. Louis, Mo.

July 12, 1944

Dear Mr. Rodale:

Since reading your fine article "Sunflower Seeds—The Forgotten Food," I took your advice and have been eating some each day for almost two months. The results are amazing. Everyone remarks on the change from a tired, harassed war worker to a healthier looking girl.

> Frances Berking
> New Hope, Pa.

June 28, 1944

Dear Mr. Rodale:

Have been eating common sunflower seed and can see considerable benefits.

Roland L. Dempsey
Fitchburg, Mass.

The following item appeared in Vol. 7, Bulletin No. 2 (1945) of the Health Education League of Portland, Ore. (27 S.E. 53rd Ave.): "SUNFLOWER SEEDS—A club member helping with the bulletin noticed that after a handful of sunflower seeds each day for a month she was able to fold the bulletins without using her glasses, which she was unable to do the month before."

I wrote to the secretary for more information and received the following reply:

May 25, 1945

Editor of *Organic Gardening* :

The Health League of Portland (sec., Mrs. Rachel Porter) told me of your letter, asking more information about my experience with sunflower seed. I am 66 years old and have always worn glasses. Have an unusually far vision, so objects near were hard to distinguish. As my health improved my glasses did not help, so I used them only for sewing or near work. I have never taken vitamins to any amount. I use about half a cup of sunflower seeds a day. I sprout some and use in salads. As I could not crack shells I

23

pour boiling water over them. Then pour water off. I eat while ironing, walking, while on bus or while reading or listening to the radio. I can at times thread a needle and sew without aid of glasses. Often go all day without glasses, which I have not been able to do for many years. I notice I have gained weight. I feel the seeds are really helping me to restore my eyesight. Our club will be glad of any more information on sunflower seed use.

I met with a bus accident, since which time I am almost constantly in pain in head, and sunflower seeds help in spite of this.

Mary Talhem
Portland, Oregon

June 10, 1945

Dear Mr. Rodale:

I suppose I have been one of the most ardent enthusiasts concerning the eating of sunflower seeds and wish to relate my experiences over the past 8 months. Despite vitamin tablets, I would come down with a sick spell every March. Last fall I discontinued with vitamins and ate sunflower seeds. This March I had no sick spell, neither had I colds during the winter. My eyes, which were causing considerable discomfort, seem much better. Whether sunflower seeds had anything to do with this I cannot say, I am just relating facts. I averaged a small handful each day.

When I ate more than this I was bothered with a rash on my forehead. This could have been caused by something else, however, and appeared only as a coincidence. Other readers may have some experience along this line by now.

I also found that there are sunflower seeds and sunflower seeds. Purchased some at a local seed store for 20¢ a pound. They were small and many were wormy. Others were purchased for 55¢ a pound from a person who claimed they were raised organically. These were large and I found none that were wormy. A few were dark and had a bad flavor (very few).

F. E. Callaghan
Baltimore, Md.

July 2, 1945

Dear Sir:

Have tried your suggestion on seeds and have found them wonderful. Have tried watermelon and cantaloupe. Can see results almost instantly on eyes, skin, etc.

M. D. Johnson
Turlock, Calif.

Dear Sir,

I believe my experience with sunflower seeds as a

remedy for eye troubles would be of interest to readers of *Prevention.*

In midsummer seven years ago, while working in my garden, I suffered a hemorrhage in my left eye. The eyeball immediately clouded up to a point where I could barely distinguish brightly lighted objects. To say I was badly scared would be an understatement; there had been no previous eye trouble, no warning whatsoever.

I immediately consulted Dr. L., an ophthalmologist, who could offer no explanation, after giving my eyes a thorough examination. He referred me to a local medical clinic for blood tests, urinalysis, tests for high blood pressure, etc., but no clue could be found.

I consulted a second ophthalmologist, Dr. J., who conducted the same tests, with the same result. He in turn referred me to an eye clinic in Chicago. Again a series of thorough tests, and again the same result. I was given the assurance that the tiny breaks in the arteries eventually would heal and the clouded eyeball would clear up. How soon? Possibly in six weeks, perhaps six months, maybe even a year. I was really frightened. Suppose I suffered the same difficulty with the right eye!

Then I remembered Mr. Rodale's little book "Sunflower Seeds, the Miracle Food," which I had read quite some time previously. Hopefully, I stopped at a Health Food store and took home a pound of seeds. The good results were immediate. The cloudy condition cleared up in three or four days. But a few strings, like cobwebs, remained for another week or ten days. Weeks later I could whip up the remnants of these strings by rotating the eyeball vigorously.

I continued the sunflower seeds for several months, and then dropped them from my diet. That proved to be a bad mistake.

A year later I had identically the same experience with the right eye. This time I did not panic, I did not go to a doctor, nor an ophthalmologist. Instead I got a goodly stock of sunflower seeds, with the same good result. I am taking no more chances. I have kept these seeds on my diet for the last six years. And I have suffered no more eye trouble, for which, at the age of 68, I am very thankful.

A one-half cupful of seeds is the main item for my breakfast almost every morning. To add flavor I nibble bits of figs or raisins, and I think this is important.

I never buy the toasted seeds; to be completely effective, they must be eaten raw. Needless to say, they must be chewed to a fine pulp, and I am not sure that children can be trusted to do so. With this in mind, let me recommend an electric seed grinder, available at any large health food dealer. This is truly a mighty fine little gadget, having the appearance of a miniature blender. Get the model with the stainless steel bowl, holding one-half cup of seeds. It will completely pulverize the seeds. The seeds may then be eaten as a cold cereal. . . .

F. W. Bassett
Beloit, Wisconsin

Chapter 4

The Anatomy of the Eye

ONE PART OF YOUR body which readily reacts to conditions of ill health or poor nourishment is the eye. The organ with which you see is the eyeball, which is actually a bulb on the end of the optic nerve leading to and from the brain. The *eyeball* is a spherically shaped organ with a section of a smaller sphere at the front—the cornea. The eyeball has three coats, the *sclera* (the white of the eye), which is protective; the *cornea,* which is muscular; and the *retina,* which is sensory—that is, full of nerves.

The *iris* is a diaphragm like that of a camera. It has a small central opening called the *pupil.* The iris is the colored part of the eye. Color pigment in the eye is often deposited some time after birth, so in babies with slate-blue eyes the color is the black pigment showing through. As the baby grows older, white, yellow, or reddish-brown pigment may be deposited on the iris, causing gray, hazel, or brown eyes. Blue eyes, then, contain less pigment than dark eyes. By means of muscular action the pupil contracts when you come into bright light or when you look at something small and near. It expands again as light grows dimmer or when you look into the distance.

The *lens* of the eye lies directly behind the pupil. It is made of layers of transparent fibers inside a clear capsule. The muscle surrounding it contracts or expands to change the shape of the lens so that it can "focus." This is called *accommodation*—that is, your eyes can accommodate themselves to distant or near objects, large or small. As one becomes older, the muscle gradually loses its elasticity, limiting the ability to see things very close or very far away. Then glasses are often necessary to do this focusing job for the lens.

Behind the lens is a cavity containing the *vitreous,* a jellylike substance, transparent and fairly solid. With age or certain diseases it becomes watery; and cells may float around in it, causing shadows to appear on the eye's retina.

The *retina,* the most important part of the eye, is filled with nerves connecting to the optic nerve and with the blood vessels which nourish the eye. These retinal vessels are the only blood vessels in the body that are visible through instruments. They indicate a great deal about the state of one's health, and diseases such as diabetes and high blood pressure can be diagnosed from the condition of these vessels. The retina also contains the center of vision, which is filled with small cones which are necessary to transmit to the brain the color and form of things we see. In dim light, the eye utilizes rods at another part of the retina for seeing. Every eye has a normal blind spot. This is at the place where the optic nerve enters the eye.

The actual process by which we see is not fully understood. However, it seems that light traveling through the rods and cones of the retina is registered by the outermost layer of the retina. There it is transformed, probably by photochemical and photoelectric means, into impulses that are carried to the optic nerve and to the brain. So the eye only receives impressions. The brain interprets these impressions into images, with color and form.

Chapter 5

Vitamins and Eyesight

VITAMIN A

MOST OF US know that lack of vitamin A causes definite eye symptoms. These are night blindness, xerophthalmia, and keratomalacia. Xerophthalmia is a dry and thickened condition of the conjunctiva, or eye tissues, which sometimes follows conjunctivitis or a disease of the tear glands. Keratomalacia is a softening of the cornea.

It is known that the normal retina and the choroid (an eye membrane) contain enormous amounts of vitamin A. Apparently vitamin A is necessary for the process that goes on inside the eye when your body moves from darkness to light or from light to darkness. So a lack of vitamin A would hinder this process.

It has been found that night blindness resulting from vitamin A deficiency may be accompanied by scotomata, that is, dark spots in the field of vision. We know that both of these conditions are directly caused by too little vitamin A and can be cured by increasing the amount of vitamin A available for the use of the body.

Often night blindness is accompanied by dryness of the cornea and the eye tissues. Triangular spots appear, silver-gray and shiny; they are called Bitot's spots, after the physician who first studied them. The area that is affected by this dryness feels gritty, as if there were grains of sand on the eyeball. Then too, as if there were a film of oil over the eye, it cannot be "wetted" by the natural fluids.

Keratomalacia is a more advanced and much more serious condition than either or both of these first two. Dryness is noticed first, followed by a softening of the cornea, which becomes gray, dull, and cloudy. Since this condition is an indication of severe vitamin A deficiency, other tissues in the body also suffer and may finally become so starved for vitamin A that the patient dies.

Vitamin A—rich carrots do help the eyesight, but too much must not be expected of them. When England pioneered radar, they thought of a scheme to allay the German's anxiety as to why the British airmen were suddenly shooting down so many German planes. They circulated a rumor that their best ace, Cat's Eye Cunningham, accomplished his results by eating tremendous amounts of carrots. The Germans adopted the idea and vast amounts of carrot were consumed but it did nothing for the acuity of the Luftwaffe pilots' eyesight.

There can be no question that vitamin A is a specific for the eye. In 119 cases of conjunctivitis among school children, a vitamin A deficiency was discovered in each. Prompt improvement and recovery were the result of giving large amounts of this vitamin (*American Journal of Diseases of Children,* July, 1941). Conjunctivitis is an inflammation of the delicate membrane that lines the eyelids. In emergency cases it is advisable to inject vitamin A, because in some persons it may not be assimilated when taken by mouth.

Foods rich with vitamin A are butter, milk, eggs, liver, and carrots. It is also found to a lesser extent in fruits and vegetables. To get enough vitamin A, it is suggested that halibut liver oil capsules be taken daily as a permanent part of everyone's diet. Vitamin A has been called the longevity vitamin. Experiments have shown that animals always live longer when this vitamin is added to their diets. As far as dosage is concerned, the usual capsule contains 5,000 units. To do any good, 3 or 4 of them should be taken per day. The toxic point would be over 40 of them per day.

VITAMIN B

It might come as a surprise that there are vitamins other than vitamin A that are necessary for the healthy functioning of the eye. The B vitamin complex, for example, is an absolute necessity; and even a partial deficiency in one or more vitamins of this complex results in serious eye symptoms. A lack of thiamin (vitamin B_1), for example, may cause pains

33

behind the eyeball. Where there is a considerable lack of it, there can occur a true paralysis of the eye muscles. Vitamin B_1 will cure neuritis of the eye.

Other B vitamins are concerned in eye health. These include riboflavin, niacin, pyridoxine, pantothenic, and folic acids. In certain forms of pellagra, for instance, giving just niacin will not cure the disease. These other members of the B family of vitamins are necessary as well. In pellagra, there is inflammation of the eyelids and loss of eyelashes, erosion of the eye tissues, and clouding of the cornea. When riboflavin is lacking in the diet, the eyelids may smart and itch, the eyes grow tired, vision may be poor and cannot be improved by glasses, it may be difficult for the individual to see in dim light, and there may be extreme sensitivity to light. This does not mean that the patient cannot stand any light at all but rather that he suffers actual physical discomfort in the presence of bright light.

Dr. V. P. Sydenstricker, of the University of Georgia, studied 47 patients, all of whom lacked riboflavin. They suffered from a variety of visual disturbances. They were sensitive to light, suffered from eyestrain that was not relieved by wearing glasses, had burning sensations in their eyes and visual fatigue, and their eyes watered easily. Six of them had cataracts. Within 24 hours after the administration of riboflavin, their symptoms began to improve. After two days, the burning sensations and the other symptoms began to disappear. Gradually, all the disorders were cured. When the riboflavin was taken away from them the symptoms gradually appeared again and once again were cured by riboflavin.

A condition known as tobacco amblyopia is a dimness or loss of vision due to poisoning by tobacco. Patients complain of blackouts, headache, and inability to read. Nearly all of them experience cold fingertips in the morning after the first cigarette. There is also a loss of the ability to see red and green colors. In every case, the patient who stops smoking soon regains full vision. In all of these cases, a vitamin B_{12} deficiency is found and injection of this vitamin brings about a cure. People who smoke strong pipe tobaccos are more likely to have the disease than are those who smoke cigarettes. Vitamin B_{12} is found in liver, also in egg yolk, and to a lesser extent in other animal products.

The safest way for the individual to ensure that he is getting every part of the vitamin B complex is to take it in the form of food supplements such as brewer's yeast, desiccated liver, wheat germ, and sunflower seeds—preferably all of them. They are of great benefit to the body's general health. It is for the individual to attempt to take invididual parts of the B complex as they occur in synthetic vitamin preparations, because serious imbalances can occur. The reason is that they exert various effects upon each other, and excesses and deficiencies may be harmful.

VITAMIN C AND THE EYES

There is abundant evidence that vitamin C is plentiful in the healthy lens of the eye. It is absent or nearly absent in the diseased lens. In the answer to a letter to the editor of the *Journal of the American Medical Association,* for December 16, 1950, we find this information: Vitamin C plays an important part in the nutrition of the eye tissues. The healthy lens is particularly rich in this vitamin, but eyes that have cataracts contain little or none.

Vitamin C is necessary for the oxygen uptake of the lens. In scurvy, there are hemorrhages of the eyelids and eye tissues; vitamin C performs an antihemorrhage function. Glaucoma and cataract are usually accompanied by very low levels of vitamin C in the lens. Extensive medical findings show that vitamin C is closely related to the health of the lens.

In the *British Medical Journal* for November 18, 1950, there is a review of 51 cases of small corneal ulcers—that is, ulcers of the cornea of the eye. About half of the patients received 1,500 milligrams of vitamin C every day, while the other half received a tablet containing nothing of medicinal value. In those who received the vitamin C there was no significant difference in the healing of the superficial ulcers, but the deep ulcers healed much more rapidly.

In *The Eye, Ear, Nose and Throat Monthly,* Vol. 31, page 79, a doctor gives his formula for preventing cataract formation and checking its progress once it is formed. He gives his patients a special diet which includes the tops of vegetables—in other words, garden greens—one pint of milk and two eggs daily. In addition, each of his patients gets vitamin supplements—chlorophyll tablets and vitamins C and A.

Cataracts is a disease of later years. And we suspect that one very good reason why they form may be that older people get out of the habit of eating eggs, leafy green vegetables, and other foods that are rich in vitamins and minerals. It is much easier and cheaper to live on white bread, soft, starchy desserts, and coffee or tea. Surveys show that older folks are especially deficient in vitamin C. They also appear to need *more* of this vitamin than younger people.

We prefer natural rose hip tablets to the synthetic ascorbic acid form of vitamin C. Rose hips are made from the berry which is the fruit of the rose plant; it is 40 times richer in vitamin C than oranges or grapefruit. It also contains other vitamins and minerals, whereas ascorbic acid is a pure chemical formula, a fragmentation which is counter to the theory of what a food should be.

Foods rich in vitamin C are green peppers, broccoli, cauliflower, water cress, kohlrabi, raw cabbage, strawberries, collards, cantaloupe, tomatoes, and fresh peas. We recommend only a moderate consumption of the citrus fruits because of their citric acid content. Overconsumption of the juices, especially, sometimes causes *pruritus ani* (itching rectum) as well as serious digestive troubles. The pulp of the fruit contains vitamin P, which is not present in the juice; vitamin P helps the body absorb vitamin C.

37

VITAMIN D

Vitamin D, the sun vitamin, is involved in cataracts. In experiments with chickens, a deficiency of it produced cloudy lenses. Vitamin D is found mainly in fish livers, which are also rich in vitamin A. Vitamin D is also found in eggs and milk. The daily taking of halibut liver oil capsules will ensure the necessary supply of A and D vitamins. There is no objectionable taste because the capsule does not dissolve until it reaches the stomach.

VITAMIN E

Vitamin E is of value to the entire body because it causes an increased oxygenation of the veins and arteries. It forces oxygen to the most inaccessible parts of the body. In Italian experiments, three patients experienced improved vision when given vitamin E over a period of three months (*Policlinico-Sezione Practica,* 58:1381, 1951).

In another Italian study, three doctors used vitamin E for ocular disturbances in 400 cases, and obtained uniformly good results. In some cases, there was improvement in visual acuity and in several there were surprising results (*Annales d'Oculistique,* 186:987-994, Nov., 1953). Dr. Evan Shute, of the Shute clinic, famous heart clinic of London, Ontario, Canada, has shown that the use of vitamin E enables new blood vessels to form.

Vitamin E assists the middle-aged eye to focus

readily, which is good news for those of us who may need glasses for close work. According to Dr. R. Seidenari, of Milan, Italy, patients over forty given vitamin E showed in tests and by their own statements that their farsightedness had improved and that they could once again read without spectacles. Dr. E. Raverdino, of Italy, used vitamin E in cases of degeneration of certain parts of the eye due to old age. He gave doses of 600-milligrams a day. In the majority of cases (except where the central vision was already completely destroyed) the results were favorable, with rapid return of vision and a reduction of the blind spot. C. Malatesta, also of Italy, reports that the results of experiments in his laboratory indicate that lack of vitamin E alone causes severe degenerative changes in the retina and the lens of the eye.

Detached retina and cataract are two rapidly increasing disorders of our time; could lack of vitamin E in the diet be partly responsible?

VITAMIN E USED AGAINST MANY EYE DISEASES

The *Summary* (Vol. 8, pages 85-93, 1956), reports on 44 cases of various ocular diseases that were treated with vitamin E for 2 to 7 months. The results were good: 7 of 14 cases of hypertensive retinopathy (inflammation of the retina), all 3 diabetic retinopathy cases, 7 of 9 cases of senile degeneration of the eyes, 1 of 4 cases of glossy dimness of the eyes, and 1 case of inflammation of the nerve behind the eyeball—all showed improvement ranging from increased vision to complete recovery. There were no side effects. It was noted, however, that glaucoma cases were not helped.

In the *Practitioner and Digest of Treatment* (July, 1956) the details of a most enlightening experiment with vitamin E are recounted. Sixteen turkey hens were reared to maturity. They were then placed in separate laying cases and fed identical synthetic diets. Half were then given vitamin E in addition, and the other half were kept on the diet deficient only in vitamin E. The hens were artificially inseminated weekly with pooled semen from the farm's toms. All care was taken to ensure that the hen turkeys ate and lived exactly alike except for the difference made by vitamin E.

The eyes of 109 embryos taken from eggs laid by the vitamin-deficient hens were examined. There were cataractlike opacities observed in 21 out of 54 vitamin E-deficient embryos. Out of 55 embryos given vitamin E supplements, only two were found to show cataractlike films over the eyes.

The usefulness of vitamin E is obviously not a figment of the imagination. There are scores of reports similar to those carried in these pages appearing in medical journals throughout the world. If added vitamin E will sometimes cure these disorders, why shouldn't a regular intake of vitamin E help to prevent them? Vitamin E is found in wheat germ and wheat germ oil, in sunflower seeds, all nuts, soybeans, and in vegetable and cereal oils and fish oils.

Chapter 6

Nutrition and Eyesight

Is THERE A CONNECTION between nutrition and eyesight? Medical research says there is. Can we eat our way into good eyesight? If you are a young child, yes. If you are older, proper nutrition can maintain the visual status quo, and it can even improve the eyesight somewhat, but more important, it can prevent serious eye disturbances that so frequently attack older persons.

Is overuse of the eyes a factor in harming vision? A physician has said, "It is almost impossible to damage the eyes by long hours of reading or sewing, even if great fatigue is experienced at those times" (Dr. J. H. Doggart, *British Medical Journal,* August 15, 1953). General health is a factor in eye health. Thus, it is important to get adequate exercise, to be outdoors sufficiently, and to observe the recognized health rules. But nutrition is the most important of all.

And what is the first rule of good nutrition? It is to

be sure that there is plenty of good protein in your diet. The word "protein" is derived from the Greek and means "of first importance."

Myopia most generally occurs in children, and this fact has provided researchers with an excellent basis for the study of nutritional effect on myopia. *The Lancet* (May, 1958) describes such a study in great detail. The eyesight of two groups of myopic children was compared. One group had 10 per cent of their normal calorie intake altered to consist of animal protein, while the control group was given no dietary advice whatsoever.

The results of the simple experiment were so conclusive that the examiners readily admitted the influence of protein on myopia. First it should be known that it is generally regarded as a rule that progressive deterioration in eyesight takes place in nearsighted people until they reach the age of twenty or so. Yet the children in this test over twelve years of age showed a definite arresting of such progress when given the protein supplement. Some of the special-diet children over twelve not only stopped getting worse but actually had their sight improved. Those children under twelve continued to deteriorate, but at only one-third the rate of those not getting the prescribed protein. And those who took the most protein deteriorated least rapidly.

Among the other findings was that an increase in myopia is greater and commoner in children who refuse to eat animal protein (meat, fish, and eggs) than in those who eat it willingly. It was also found that myopic children whose eyes are deteriorating eat less food, yet gain more weight, than normally sighted children. Obviously the myopics have disorders in metabolism which do not allow for the proper use of the food they eat. Could this be due to a lack of food-processing enzymes found in the protein foods they refuse to consume? Are you heading off the possibility of nearsightedness in your children by including plenty of protein in their diet?

One should eat plenty of the protective foods— meats, eggs, green leafy vegetables, yellow vegetables and fruits (for vitamin A), and all kinds of fresh vegetables and fruits (for vitamin B and C). And we can't stress too strongly how necessary it is to eat fruits and vegetables *raw* whenever possible. Heat and exposure to light and air are not friendly to B vitamins and vitamin C. So the more cooking, shredding, and storing you put your foods through before eating them, the less of these vitamins you will have. If you live in the North, it is hardly possible to get enough vitamin D in the winter unless you supplement your diet with fish liver oils. Never take synthetic vitamin D.

Fish liver oils contain larger amounts of vitamin A than any other food, so they are, we think, an absolute necessity for eye health, especially if you aren't willing to make a conscious effort to eat lots of yellow vegetables such as carrots and sweet potatoes. The B vitamins are those neglected orphans, so scarce in our present-day diets which include so much white bread, cake, and refined cereals. Eat lots of fresh

43

vegetables and fruits and organ meats, such as liver and kidney, if you want to get even a smattering of the B vitamins you need. In addition, we strongly suggest supplementing your diet with desiccated liver or brewer's yeast for those extra B vitamins. Don't take synthetics, which may contain only one or only a few of the B vitamins. You must have them all, for they work together in your body's chemistry; and if you are short of one, you are almost certain to be deficient in others, too. Brewer's yeast and desiccated liver contain them all.

Just a few more cautions on vitamin C. Over and over again it has been brought to our attention that aging goes hand in hand with vitamin C deficiency. Maybe we need more vitamin C as we grow older. Perhaps we just gradually stop eating vitamin C-rich foods after middle age. At any rate, cataract, along with so many other diseases of old age, is closely related to vitamin C deficiency. Is there any logical reason to look forward to an old age clouded by cataract, when all kinds of vitamin C-rich foods are available to use the year round? We think not. And this is why we dwell so persistently on the importance of vitamin C in our diets. Don't shove aside that bit of parsley on your plate. Parsley is rich in vitamin C. Eat it by the handful every day. Buy watercress whenever you can find it, or grow your own if you live in the country. Get used to the idea of whopping big tossed salads that are green with watercress, endive, raw spinach, and any other greens you can find. Bleached vegetables have few vitamins. Shun them.

And finally, because we are sure you are not getting enough vitamin C every day of your life, take rose hips as a food supplement. They contain more vitamin C than any other food and are rich in vitamins A, E, K, and B as well. For nibbling between meals, you won't find anything more delicious or better for your eyes than sunflower seeds. Here's health to your eyes!

SUGAR

There are other factors in nutrition that should be considered relative to vision. There is hardly any other organ of the body that is so dependent on good blood chemistry as the eye. The blood which feeds this organ should be as close to physiological perfection as possible. We should, therefore, avoid anything that distorts it. The overuse of sugar is the greatest offender in this respect. It causes a distortion of the calcium-phosphorus relationship of the blood. It also produces a condition of *low* blood sugar, strange as this might seem. Teenagers are now more frequently fitted with glasses than those of previous eras; and in connection with this, we cannot overlook their jitterbug diet, with its accent on candy, ice cream, cakes, pastries, soft drinks, etc. If sugar can cause cavities in the teeth, what is its effect on other, more delicate organs? A note of caution is called for in the use of this category of food.

CALCIUM

Dr. A. Huber has written a long article (*Ophthalmologia,* October, 1948) describing how he found calcium to be an effective means of clearing stubborn cases of inflammation of the pigmented layer of the eye, stating that a great amount of corroborative material has been accumulating in the medical literature. He quotes the work of six physicians who obtained the same results. He quotes, also, the work of other physicians who obtained results with calcium in certain kinds of conjunctivitis and in photophobia, which is an intolerance of the eye to light. He found it valuable also in excessive winking and in watering of the eye. Then he states, "The numerous reports of the efficacy of calcium therapy for the eye are now opposed, not only by the skepticism of strict scientific thought, but also by the hesitant attitude of many a practitioner."

In my reading of medical literature, and I subscribe to 30 medical journals, I find such skepticism quite general in the medical profession's attitude toward the use of nutritional measures to combat and prevent disease. It is probably due to the training the medical student is given. He spends 99 per cent of his curricular time in studying the use of drugs and surgery. Nutrition is still the stepchild of the medical sciences.

Milk is not the best food for obtaining calcium. There is evidence that pasteurization does something to the calcium in it that makes much of it unavailable to the human body. I don't say *not* to pasteurize milk, but if you are going to drink it with a feeling that you are getting calcium, you may wake up some fine day and find yourself calcium deficient. Bone meal tablets are a sure way of getting needed calcium. Their effect in preventing cavities of the teeth is nothing short of sensational.

So much for specific elements of nutrition and their effect on the eye. But one word of caution: Many physicians are against the use of vitamins except in emergency situations. They say, "Get your vitamins with your knife and fork"; but this is impossible, as can be seen by the extent of vitamin deficiencies prevailing in the public. There is an alarming decline in soil fertility that is reducing the nutritional quality of our food. There is much destruction of vitamins in the processing of food in the factories. Kitchen practices such as cooking, storing, soaking, and paring take much out of food. Natural vitamins and minerals must be taken daily to restore that part of the food of which we are being robbed in so many ways by the system of food production that our civilization forces upon us.

SOFT DRINKS

I have discussed briefly the possible effect of sugar on the eyes. May I speak for a moment or two about the effect of soft drinks on our vision? According to Dr. Hunter H. Turner, writing in the *Pennsylvania Medical Journal* (May, 1944), one of the predisposing causes of myopia, or nearsightedness, is the drinking of carbonated beverages. He states his belief that the carbonic acid they contain is the eye's worst enemy and attributes the alarming increase in myopia cases to "the pernicious guzzling of carbonated beverages by young children today."

In the stomach, he says, carbonated drinks break down into their basic ingredients of water and carbon dioxide, which go to every part of the body. In the eye, it produces a chronic waterlogging of important structures. An abnormal amount of fluid in the tissues of the white of the eye causes a constriction of the vessels that traverse it and result in their congestion.

Yet medical journals regularly accept the advertisements of soft drink manufacturers. Here is a typical statement appearing in a recent ad: "The 'catalyst' of everybody's love of the carbonated soft drink is CO_2!" CO_2 is carbon dioxide, the very thing that should make the medical journal violently refuse such an advertisement.

CONCLUSION

I have presented a great deal of data showing a direct connection between vitamins and minerals and the eyes, and that where nutrition went down, so did the ability to see. Does this hold any hope for adults, that is, to enable them to rid themselves of their glasses? I do not claim that. It can, however, prevent the onset of the terrible scourges of cataract, glaucoma, and senile blindness. It might also prevent the eyesight from further deterioration and assure full use of the eyes into a healthy old age. It is part of the battle against general senility.

It is with children that the greatest hope lies. There the possibilities are far-reaching. There can be no question that with a strong program to encourage proper nutrition, their eyesight can be preserved in all the strength conferred upon it at birth. In this regard, the Bausch and Lomb Optical Company has said, "As enzymes control all our metabolic processes and enzymes are composed of vitamins (or hormones or both), together with minerals and specific proteins, there is opportunity during the constructive stages of life to improve the condition of the eye through enhancing the nutritive values of the diet" (*Optical Developments*, February, 1957).

Such enhancement of the nutritive values of the diet can begin in the home, but the schools can be a powerful influence also in teaching children about these nutritional practices that are harmful to the eyes. I would like to see developed an "eyesight" tablet made up of halibut liver oil for vitamin C, vitamin E, bone meal, and rutin, to be given daily to children in the schools. As part of the campaign, there could be large, blown-up photographs in the corridors of schools, of a goose wearing horn-rimmed glasses, with the caption, "Do you too want to be a four-eyed goose?"

Such a nutritional program would not only be conducive to an improvement in the general level of the country's vision but also would build the health of the body generally. We must get the schools to make a thorough investigation of the facts enumerated in this discussion and take a strong hand toward adopting them into school health programs.

REFINED FOOD, ENEMY OF VISION

The 268 natives of Tristan da Cunha, an island in the South Atlantic Ocean, had perfect teeth when examined by a Norwegian survey team in 1937. Then a British Navy Canteen was opened and began selling canned goods, biscuits, sugar, coffee, tea, cocoa, beer, and other alcoholic drinks. Mothers began feeding their babies sweetened condensed milk instead of nursing them. By 1961, the Islanders were suffering from cavities and much gum disease. Even more widespread, however, was the incidence of eye disorders: cataracts, glaucoma, nearsightedness, and infectious ailments.

The "slow infiltration of civilization" is responsible for this sad deterioration of health, according to a new book, *Culture, Race, Climate and Eye Disease* by Ida Mann, an Australian ophthalmologist and research scientist. From an extensive study of peoples the world over, Dr. Mann has discovered that wherever Western man introduces his nutritional habits, the eye health and general clinical status of the "contaminated" people are considerably worsened.

Dr. Mann's homeland, Western Australia, is pointed to as an excellent illustration of the effects of different nutritional habits upon eye health. From her clinical practice, Dr. Mann has observed that eye ailments are common among the "civilized" white people but rare among the primitive tribes of aborigines. She attributes much of the white natives' ulcerated corneas, cataracts, squint, and defective vision to tobacco, alcohol, and nutritional deficiency in general.

Australian patients with severe opacity of the cornea, she has found, have usually been living on black tea, white bread, jam, overcooked vegetables, and canned goods. Such a diet leads surely to deficiency in riboflavin (vitamin B_2), a cause of major eye disturbances. In many cases Dr. Mann has been able to bring about dramatic recovery, however, with intramuscular injections of this vitamin.

It is not difficult to see why Western Australia is called "the land of sin, sand, sorrow, and sore eyes." How could it be otherwise when the common diet is uniformly deficient in vitamin B_2? Some of the recognized signs of B_2 deficiency are bloodshot eyes, conjunctivitis (eyelid inflammation), sandy lids, and itching, burning, and watering.

Like the inhabitants of Tristan da Cunha, the Western Australians, by turning to refined foods, are depriving themselves of nutrition that is essential to health. The aborigines of the same region, however, rarely, if ever, suffer from nutritional deficiency and have uniformly excellent eyes.

Aborigines are rarely eye patients unless they have come into contact with the white Western Australi-

51

ans. They are nomads who hunt their food in the desert, thriving on kangaroo, lizard, snake, fish, and crocodile meat. They have also been observed to eat up to 8 pounds of meat a day. Berries, grass seed, roots, and wild fruits, all sources of vitamins C and E, fill out their nutritional needs.

A survey discovered that even when the tribe went for prolonged periods without food, there were "no eye signs of deficiency disease, and the only suggestive finding was of early scurvy (spongy gums) in five children boarding at a mission and eating European food (white bread and tinned food)."

When aborigines do contact an infectious eye ailment, it is of a mild type. No case of marginal blepharitis, an eyelid infection widespread among whites, has been reported among the tribesmen, "unless they are assimilated." Dr. Mann mourns the fact that the physically and nutritionally fit aborigines are being forced to assimilate into the general population.

She notes, "As soon as these people come in contact with Western culture they begin to abandon their natural habits. Raw flour and water look much like milk and are fed to babies who also like refined sugar, so one sees occasionally on the stations some indications of kwashiorkor (protein-calorie deficiency disease), though this is rare, and never seen in the bush. Teeth suffer most from introduction to European food."

The situation is similar in other countries where natives are subjected to Western influence, accord-

52

ing to Dr. Mann. In Alaska, eye disease and other "illnesses are all more accentuated where the people are living in contact with Caucasian settlers." The Alaskan's eye ailments, low life expectancy, and high mortality rate are largely due to "overcrowding, introduction of the diseases of civilization," and "a strangely unbalanced diet" (seal meat, fish, fat, and little vitamin C). And in Brazil, "disease diminished with decreased contact with white men."

Yet, one race cannot be considered directly responsible for lowering the health of another. Even Negroes who live in different environments show different health levels. Dr. Mann notes that color blindness is only 1.86 per cent among Bantu (African) males, but "among the American Negro it has risen to 3.5 per cent."

Among other African tribes there is much eye disease, and it occurs where protein and the B and C vitamins are lacking in the diet. Such tribes, of course, are those that have come closely into contact with European civilization and have taken on the food preferences of the European.

"India is a land of eye disease," writes Dr. Mann, noting that within one year there were 88,370 eye operations and 465,621 new eye patients. Protein intake is minimal in India because some religions ban meat and others ban all protein in times of illness. Rice has long been considered the complete food by the villagers, who have stayed away from green vegetables and unrefined sugar because "they had no prestige appeal." The Jains (members of one religious sect), who drink large quantities of milk, also have a high incidence of glaucoma. Blindness, cataracts and infectious eye disorders are common throughout India.

Dr. Mann has tried to determine the "influence of diet, climate, cultural habits, race and heredity on the incidence and nature of disease." All these factors play a part in the development of specific ills, but nutritional habits stand out above the others.

While out-and-out starvation plays a role in the causation of eye disease, it is a strange fact that countries in which food is scarce seem to have better eye health than countries like ours, where food is abundant. Throughout the world, sadly enough, man is almost always uniformly ignorant of the principles of good nutrition. Given a choice, he invariably chooses the foods that are worst for him: sugar, white bread, sweet cakes, and all the other well-known nutritional vices. Fortunate are those whose choices are limited to fresh, unrefined natural foods. Where there is too much choice, as in the United States, it is apparent that instinct cannot be relied upon; everything must be learned about our nutritional needs.

Chapter 7

Smoke Gets in Your Eyes

THE EYES OF THE HUNZUKUTS

IN 1948 I WROTE a book, *The Healthy Hunzas,* about a race that is perhaps the healthiest in the world. They number about 25,000 people at the northern-most region of India, next to Tibet. They do not get cancer, diabetes, or appendicitis; they have stalwart bodies. But there is one condition that is unhappily prevalent among them, and that is an affliction of the eyes in the form of glaucoma, cataracts, and granulated lids. Major General Sir Robert McCarrison, M.D., Director of the India Nutrition Research Laboratories, Coonoor, India, said that it was due to the manner in which they make fires in their homes. The Hunzukut's house has two rooms, a smaller one in which supplies are kept and a room in which the entire family—usually two or three families—lives, eats, and sleeps. The houses of neighboring races, who are far below the Hunzas in general intelligence, as a rule consist of only one squalid room.

The Hunzukut's living room is made of stone plastered over with mud. The floor is of hard, rammed earth of the consistency of stone. On one side of the room is a large dais used by the men for sitting and sleeping and made of stones and mud. On the other side there is a dais for the women. Cupboards are built in at the side of the dais, but there are no chairs. Furnishings are at an irreducible minimum. There are no windows.

In the center of the room is a hearth consisting of a shallow, square hole dug below the ground level and framed with stone. Above this, in the ceiling, is the smoke hole, an aperture about two or three feet square, which is the only egress for the smoke from the open fire below. Fuel is cruelly scarce in this poverty-stricken mountain region of Northern Asia. A small amount of firewood made into an open fire on the sunken dirt hearth heats up quickly, and it throws its warmth farther than a metal stove does. Much fuel would have to be squandered to heat up a stove. The fumes twirl and eddy about, though, tormenting the occupants and irritating their eyes.

In Hunza the shortage of firewood is so great that even during the coldest days of winter, fires are made only to cook meals. The family then gathers around the warm ashes to get the benefit of the last bit of heat from the dying embers. In the winter the cold is so severe that for a period of about two months the entire family is house-bound. The Hunzukuts refer to this period as the Great Cold.

Even so, the Hunza living rooms are not fouled up with smoke as badly as the rooms of neighboring peoples, some of whom permit the smoke to escape from mere chinks in the roof. But the condition is bad enough to make the average Hunzukut easily susceptible to eye diseases such as glaucoma and cataracts.

The books written by travelers and explorers who have journeyed through these regions are replete with dramatic instances showing how general this condition is. E. F. Knight, in *Where Three Empires Meet,* says:

"We selected the biggest hut, where we found a group of coolies squatting round a large fire in the middle of the mud floor. The only firewood procurable was that of the dwarf birch, which here covers the hillsides; the smoke of this is peculiarly suffocating and irritating to the eyes, and as there were few orifices in the roofs and walls to allow its escape, we were kept weeping and coughing till bedtime."

Ella K. Maillart, in *Forbidden Journey,* describes how the ethnographer Bokkenkamp escaped from a jail at Hami, in China. In these sparsely inhabited northern regions the natives look to passing white travelers for medical help, as they always seem to be amply stocked with medical supplies for the needs of their trip. Miss Maillart states:

"His jailer had sore eyes. Bokkenkamp poured some drops inside the eyelids for him, and then

57

blindfolding him, told him he would lose his sight unless he remained in darkness for three days!" Thus he was able to escape.

THE AMERICAN INDIAN

Trachoma, another eye disease, affects more than 500 million persons, or roughly about one-quarter of the world's population. The *Newsweek* issue of February 5, 1940, is responsible for this assertion. The United States, however, has only 60,000 cases, the American Indian and people living in the Southern hill country being most affected. In connection with its cause, says *Newsweek*, "Public-health officials . . . believe there may be other as-yet-undiscovered factors—including the eye-straining effect of smoke from open fires in log cabins." Those of you who love a roaring, open log fire, look to the efficiency of your fireplace. Also be aware that the wood from conifers gives off more irritating smoke than other woods.

The American Indians are afflicted with these eye ailments because of inadequate ventilation of their homes. Excessive group smoking in confined spaces is a weighty factor. A notable example is a peyote meeting among the Sioux Indians. Peyote is a cactus grown in Mexico, which causes intoxication and produces visions when eaten; it also induces sensuousness. In recent years, over 100,000 American Indians have founded a new religion based on the eating of peyote, to which they give a religious significance. But it is in the same class as cocaine, heroin, marihuana, morphine, and opium, a dope pure and simple. Meetings begin on Saturday evening and last all night. Twenty or more peyote eaters gather in a tent or a small log cabin, where they sit on the floor in a circle. Thick tobacco smoke eddies over their coal black hair and dark brown faces. Is it any wonder, then, that so many Indians are developing trachoma? On a recent trip to Arizona and New Mexico I saw many Navajo Indian *hogans,* windowless little one-room log cabins with slits in the roof from which the smoke escapes. Cases are on record of the tobacco-smoke-filled atmosphere of a room causing the death of infants.

MY PERSONAL EYE HISTORY

When I was a young man of about twenty-six, an embarrassing blink developed in my eyes. As the president of a concern manufacturing electric wiring devices and employing over a hundred persons, I regarded this as an awkward complication. I went to an eye, ear, nose, and throat doctor whose speciality was the extracting of tonsils, and he ran true to form. He solemnly pronounced that my affliction was caused by diseased tonsils. I distinctly recall the positive manner in which he delivered this pronouncement. I submitted to the operation, but unfortunately the blinks persisted.

An old eye-doctor friend of mine whom I usually consulted when I needed a change of spectacles was the head of the eye department of one of New York's finest hospitals. An authority in medical circles, he had a charming personality and gave a delightful dissertation on life and philosophy with every prescription. He saw nothing organically or functionally wrong, so he suggested that I visit a certain nerve specialist—today we would call him a psychiatrist. He put me through psychoanalysis at the rate of $25 a visit. At that time psychiatrists were practically supported by old, crotchety millionaires who had an abundance of money and who wanted someone to listen to their troubles.

Psychiatrists often effect miraculous cures by getting hold of some red herring which has left a smear on the patient's childhood. The doctor sometimes routs the plaguey thing out of the nettles of the subconscious by bringing it strongly into the limelight. I can't remember everything I told him, but I do recall that he was seeking items that contained an element of frustration. Whenever I mentioned bits of happenings showing that I was thwarted, baffled, balked, or hindered in any way, the professor's ears would stand out exuberantly and his penciled hand would race across his pad.

He was keenly interested in my Aunt Zelda, who was a daily visitor at our house, so I told him about an episode which was quite frustrating. When I studied biology at high school I learned about the metamorphosis of the frog: how it began life as a tadpole, how it lost its tail and legs gradually, and how after a while it became an adult frog.

Aunt Zelda was a strong character who had come

from the old country. When I told her these simple facts she did not react at all in a manner to my liking. "What kind of rubbish are you giving me?" she snorted. "Didn't I see in Europe frogs getting born by the thousands, right before my very eyes? What kind of teachers do you have?"

"All right, Aunty, I will show you."

So I got an aquarium and a few tadpoles, and Aunt Zelda came every day to keep a sharp lookout and to see that I did not palm anything off on her.

One day I said, "Look, Aunty, do you see that tadpole's tail? It's getting shorter."

"Where is it getting shorter?"

She wouldn't acknowledge anything until the tiny legs started to develop. Then she made sounds showing that she was extremely interested and that it was a wonderful miracle she was witnessing. I was as proud as Einstein on the day he came face to face with relativity. The metamorphic process continued. Aunt Zelda marveled and "tsk, tsked." Then came the payoff. There they were one day, a half-dozen full-fledged jumpy frogs hopping about the tank.

"So you see, Aunty, frogs *do* start as tadpoles," I lectured, with the condescending air of a professor of zoology. Evidently I had completely mistaken Aunt Zelda's reactions to the experiment; she was far from understanding.

"These are American frogs," she argued. "In Europe we don't have such monkey business. There, when a frog is born, he's a frog right away, and no nonsense about it. I have seen it with my own eyes."

61

If that wasn't frustration then I'm the Swedish ambassador's aunt.

The nerve specialist, an extremely dignified man, burst out laughing. I can distinctly recall this phase of the examination, but he did not seem to attach any frustrational importance to the experience. I blinked through ten visits, and the doctor (who rarely uttered a word, but kept recording as if he were a court stenographer) soon began to make me feel that I was really going into a decline. These cozy monologues were too one-sided: his part of the conversation was twenty-five dollars, and see me next Tuesday." I understand that the science of psychoanalysis has been marching forward and that today the doctor and patient actually conduct a two-way conversation, especially at the beginning. I slowly arrived at the conclusion that I needed psychiatry like a hole in the head, so by prearrangement I did not show up one Tuesday—$250 gone and the blinks about as fluttery as ever.

About a year later I undertook matrimony and within a month my eye affliction cleared up as if by magic. Naturally, I set to thinking to ascertain the cause of this extraordinary occurrence, to find out the relationship between marriage and eyes that did not blink. As a young man I was studiously inclined and had shunned dance halls and night clubs. But at the age of twenty-six, with a fat income at my command, friends and night clubs had begun to beckon. I soon was a confirmed night club habitué, and it was quite common for me to be out gallivanting till four in the morning. The pernicious combination of late hours and eye irritation from the smoke-laden atmosphere which generally befogs night clubs must have been at the bottom of my eye complaint.

Alcoholic liquors held no appeal for me. I did the very minimum of drinking that drinking companions would tolerate. It was most assuredly the smoke and insufficient sleep that had robbed my eyes of needed rest and the soothing action of closed lids. Here were three wise men—the specialist, the eye doctor, and the psychiatrist—all trained along technical lines, probing for functional, medically recognized symptoms. To pry into the simple, day-by-day habits of a person was beneath their professional dignity. The eye doctor is especially to blame since, in the first place, he specialized in eyes, and second, he evinced a propensity for indulging in pleasant conversation with his patients. Had he left Aristotle out of his delightful discourses and stuck more to J. I. Rodale, he might have found an interesting solution to a stubborn case.

SMOKY ROOMS

Recently I met an old friend who told me a sad story about his eyes. He was beginning to have trouble with them, and the symptoms sounded like cataracts. He had been to many physicians and had submitted to dozens of examinations, but none of them could unearth any logical reason why his eyes should be troubling him. As he narrated his story, I did some quick thinking. This man was an inveterate card player. I could picture him in a foul, smoke-laden atmosphere for hours several times each week, hunched over his cards, the proverbial cigar always in his mouth. So I said to him, "John, you like playing cards, don't you?" His reply was, "Do I? Why, twice a week a bunch of us boys hire a room at a hotel, lock ourselves in, and play until four or five in the morning." And no doubt the filthy smoke could be cut with a knife. I was certain that his eye affliction was caused by the constant irritation of the foul cigar smoke, and told him so. But since it sounded unprofessional, he wasn't impressed.

Newspapermen like to gather in hotel rooms and play cards in a smoke-filled atmosphere. Heywood Broun, along with Howard Lindsay, Russel Crouse, Marc Connelly, Arthur Kober, and F.P.A. were part of a card playing group called the *Thanatopsis Literary and Inside Straight Club.* It was nothing more than a weekly poker game that at times had been known to run over 30 hours. Once when Heywood Broun was on a newspaper strike, he urged that the game be kept going till 10 A.M. so he could make his picket line. Sometimes members of the group have games going simultaneously in New York and Hollywood, and Lindsay is known to have said on one occasion, "With luck and a plane I can make both games in one week." It is too bad that separate statistics of eye diseases are not kept for journalists, especially columnists.

There is the case of another acquaintance, a man of about seventy, who owns many properties. I noticed his sign in an empty store window, offering the place for rent. He gave two telephone numbers where he could be reached. Mr. X had a serious case of glaucoma and had been to many expensive specialists, but he had finally become resigned to a cheerless future. He had refused to be operated upon, and his eyes were in miserable condition. I had some business to transact with him, so I called one telephone number. He was out. I then called the other number, and it turned out to be the Owls Club. Imagine! He spent so much time there that he actually used the place as an office. I found him playing cards in a room thick with tobacco smoke, and unless I am greatly mistaken his condition is due to probably thirty or forty years of hanging around in a smoke-laden atmosphere.

Coming into an occasional smoke-filled room will do very little harm to the eyes. Nature has given us such fine organs in our bodies. But when it is done every few days, the eyes may eventually rebel. Lodge meetings are notorious offenders in connection with tobacco smoke, and many Americans are passionately addicted to the lodge habit. We are a nation of joiners. The average American no doubt belongs to three or four lodges or societies of one sort or another. In a recent Philadelphia mayoralty campaign the manager of one of the candidates made much of the fact that his man swore allegiance to 39 different lodges and organizations. He severely trounced his unfortunate opponent, who could muster membership in only 25.

Once on a train trip, I was passing a private Pullman compartment, when the door suddenly opened and four fine-looking American businessmen emerged. The compartment was exceedingly small, and it was practically solid with smoke. I had a chance to analyze carefully the fact of the first man coming out and noted his bloodshot eyes. Dollars to doughnuts he has an eye condition due to nothing more than tobacco smoke. Now, here were intelligent human beings who are engaged in enterprises which require shrewdness; but they didn't have sense enough to know that they were doing themselves irreparable harm by being cooped up in such a small room filled with tobacco smoke.

Air conditioning in night clubs is becoming more or less general. This movement should spread to take in the conditioning of lodge meeting rooms and specially designated card-playing rooms in hotels. In modern air conditioning, the air of a room is continually removed, along with the smoke that is in it, so one can appreciate its benefit to the eyes. If the medical profession would realize the tremendous health value of air conditioning certain public places, it would take a hand in helping to make rooms where crowds gather safe for the eyes. Now if some way could be found to give the Hunzas plenty of fuel so that they could use chimneys and normal stoves, perhaps their health could be increased to a perfect score.

Chapter 8

Tobacco Hurts the Eyes

By H. S. Hedges, M.D.
Charlottesville, Va.

Amid all the heated controversy as to the relation between lung cancer and cigarettes, I find practically nothing about the damage to eyesight; but,
frankly, if the findings in my small-town practice are
any indication of the possible results to our smokers
all over the country, there must be thousands of men
(and women, too) who are on the way to industrial
blindness if they keep on long enough.

Of course, we all know that thousands and thousands of people smoke all their lives with no apparent
trouble except the formation of a vicious drug addic-
tion, which is *very* hard to overcome. Not long ago
a big, strong man came into my office with the story
that "when driving, often everything goes black
before me." His eyes showed typical, early tobacco
trouble, and I begged him to stop smoking. He came
in again a few days ago, telling me "It was the hard-
est thing I ever had to do, but I haven't had a black-
out since."

In these tobacco eyes, the first symptom is usually

premature presbyopia (the condition most middleaged people develop in which you must hold reading matter rather far from the eyes to be able to focus on it). A strong man of thirty-eight with perfect distant vision came complaining of headache on close work and utter inability to read at all. He could read with a glass for a person 10 years older than he was. He stopped his cigarettes short and in less than three weeks all of his headaches were gone and he reads as well as anyone without a glass.

We see this condition so often among our women. They have not been smoking long enough to have developed the late nerve changes, but the premature presbyopia is my concern. Nearly all of them also complain of cold fingertips in the morning, after the first cigarette. In many of these women, if you get them quite early in the morning, place a delicate thermometer between fingertips, let them smoke one cigarette and you can measure definite fall of temperature. Among many, the flow of blood in the arterioles will fall 30 per cent; in men, about 10 per cent. And please tell me, if the arterioles of the fingers are so affected, why cannot the little vessels of the heart show the same trouble? I am told that they are controlled by a different nerve supply.

The next commonest symptom is a central loss of red and green. [Dr. Hedges is speaking of color blindness.] The test is easily made. Fix a deep red circle about one-quarter of an inch in diameter on the end of a small rod. Sit facing your patient about 4 feet away, close one of his eyes and with the other let him look straight into one of yours. Now, move the little circle slowly before his eye as he fixes yours. If the color fades in the very center of the field but remains clear in the periphery (around the edges), you may be sure that trouble is starting; and later on, all central red and green will be lost. By the time this has come about, the central distant vision is failing fast; and in some, it will be down to 20/200 (Industrial Blindness). Very marked changes will have developed in the nerve head, the whole of this area carrying the papillomacular bundle, becoming a dirty gray. Fortunately, however, if these patients will really stop all use of tobacco, most of them will make an excellent recovery.

This spring a cigarette smoker came in, the picture of despair, a man about fifty who had been a truck driver. "Doctor, my eyes have failed so that I have lost my job; I can't see well enough to do any work, I have a family to care for, and I have nothing."

Vision 20/200, unimproved with glasses (Industrial Blindness). To make a long story short, he had typical tobacco eyes. I begged him to stop his cigarettes and he said he would. He came in again a few weeks ago —the happiest looking man I have seen in a long time. "Doctor, my sight has all come back," (it tested normal) "and I have the best job I ever had."

We could give you dozens of case reports, but the best description of tobacco amblyopia that I know is found in Dr. DeSchweinitz' *Toxic Amblyopia,* published by Lea Brothers, in 1896. The earliest I can find is by Beer, 1792 and the next by the great Scot

MacKenzie in 1832. So, you see, the trouble has been known for a long time, but many still know nothing about it. One of the scientists on the Tobacco Investigating Committee wrote me he "had never heard of such a thing."

As to the much-publicized filters, while some of them doubtless remove some of the tar, they have very little effect on the unburned nicotine in the smoke. Nicotine, however, is very soluble in water, so one brand carries a damp sponge. The water in this will absorb most of the nicotine. I had a patient who needed to stop smoking, but would not; so I bought him a pack of the above type. Result: "I might as well not smoke at all." It is the nicotine that the old addict craves, and only a cigarette carrying the full percentage of the drug will or can "satisfy."

(Reprinted by permission of
The Medical Times, October, 1957)

AMBLYOPIA AND VITAMIN B$_{12}$

According to the medical journal, *The Lancet* (August 9, 1958), in amblyopia there is usually a deficiency of Vitamin B$_{12}$. Investigators have discovered that recovery from amblyopia is practically assured when this vitamin is administered. Previously, in order to effect the cure, the patient had to give up smoking. From this, it would seem that B vitamins are used up when a person smokes. (There is also medical evidence that smoking destroys Vitamin C in the body.)

70

Chapter 9

Cataracts

WHAT IS CATARACT?

A CATARACT IS A disorder of the lens of the eye, generally spoken of as a "degenerative disorder"; that is, it results from things wearing out and breaking down, rather than from "catching something" or being injured.

In the eye with a cataract, the lens becomes opaque, like a misty or fogged windowglass. The lens is that part of the eye which gathers the rays of light and focuses them on the nerve endings behind it. Apparently what happens in cataract is that cells die or are damaged, turning white in the process. Clusters of these white cells are what you see in the eye with the fully advanced cataract. A cataract is not a "growth"—that is, it is not in the same class with tumors. It does not represent cells growing abnormally. It appears rather to represent cells dying off and becoming useless.

IS THERE MORE THAN ONE KIND OF CATARACT?

Yes, there are several. *Senile* cataract is the commonest—the one most people mean then they speak of cataract. The word "senile" is used here because this kind of cataract usually afflicts people who are advanced in age, although, like gray hair and wrinkles, it can occur in quite young persons as well.

Congenital cataract occurs in babies at birth. *Diabetic* cataract sometimes afflicts diabetics of any age; it is believed to go along with degenerative changes in blood vessels that also occur in diabetics.

DOES CATARACT CAUSE BLINDNESS?

It does. It is the first and most important cause of blindness in this country today. It is estimated that 49,000 Americans are sightless because of cataract. This does not mean, of course, that everyone who gets a cataract will become blind; quite the contrary is true. Modern surgery can remove the lens of the eye on which the cataract is spread, replacing it with a powerful lens in spectacles. The patient then can see so long as he has his glasses on. When the cataract is fully developed, light cannot pass through the opacity, so there is no way for an individual with a fully developed cataract to see as long as the cataract remains on his lens.

IS THE OPERATION FOR CATARACT PAINFUL AND RISKY?

No. It seems that the biggest hazard is the patient's frame of mind. He may have worked himself into such a state of dread and anxiety that it takes him a long time to recover his peace of mind after the operation. But the time in the hospital is, it seems, far pleasanter than for most operations. Generally a local anesthesia is given so that the discomforts of general anesthesia are avoided. The percentage of failures is apparently very low. If there are no other complications, there is every chance that the patient will be able to see quite well after the operation is over and the new lenses have been made.

We are not, of course, enthusiastic about surgery. We believe that cataracts can be prevented by proper diet and care of the eyes. But, if one has *not* prevented the cataract and is in imminent danger of losing his sight, it does seem sensible to think calmly and reasonably about an operation.

WHAT CAUSES CATARACT?

We do not know. Oh, of course, we do know of some circumstances that appear to be related to the formation of cataracts. Men who work in extremely high temperatures, exposed to the blasting heat of great furnaces, are especially susceptible to cataracts, and it is assumed that these cataracts are occupational diseases.

73

Again, dinitrophenol is a drug taken as a reducing aid. It increases the basal metabolism rate so that the patient can lose weight. Cataracts are quite common, we are told, among women past forty who have taken this drug to reduce. And cataracts can be produced in animals by giving them this drug. (Isn't it amazing that women would take such a dangerous drug and risk blindness rather than reducing sensibly?)

We know, too, that smoke may have a lot to do with causing cataracts—both cigarette smoke and smoke from fires. The Hunzas, as we noted before, a perfectly healthy nation otherwise, suffer from eye disorders because the arrangement of their houses does not leave much room for the smoke from their fires to escape. When one considers the thick pall of tobacco smoke in which many of us pass our days (whether we smoke ourselves or just spend our time with those who do), it is not surprising that cataracts are so common, since the tobacco smoke is highly irritating to the eyes.

It has also been suggested that long exposure to bright sunlight may have something to do with producing cataracts, for people living in India are especially susceptible to them. And rural folks who work outside a lot seem to have more than those who work indoors. However, we must not forget that other things may be responsible as well. One researcher tells us that the average cataract patient in India is suffering from a number of different deficiency diseases. Perhaps the cataract is just one of these.

Hardening is a general tendency of the aging

body, according to one authority. Cataract is another manifestation of this tendency, he says. The blood vessels harden, the muscles become stiff, the skin becomes horny. And the lens of the eye becomes opaque, says he. It's just another indication of old age and nothing can be done about it. This does not, of course, explain either the many young people with cataracts, nor yet the babies who are born with cataracts.

We at *Prevention* magazine believe that the cause of cataracts is faulty nutrition, and a lot more will be said in support of this theory in Chapter 10. In doing research for this chapter we were astonished to find that many, many scientists and physicians admit that a cataract is a result of poor nutrition, but very few suggest correcting or preventing it by diet!

Before birth, blood is brought to the human lens by a blood vessel which withers away before the baby is born. So the lens, which is bathed in the fluid of the eye, has no way of getting nourishment except from that fluid. Hence it cannot rebuild itself as well as tissues in other parts of the body can, well nourished as they are with food brought by the blood. It gradually becomes brittle and inelastic. The center of the lens gets less nourishment than the edges, so generally the cataract starts in the center and spreads out gradually.

HOW CAN I TELL WHETHER OR NOT I HAVE A CATARACT?

You can't, actually. Many cataracts go undetected by the individuals who have them until they begin to interfere with vision. If you notice any peculiarity of vision it would be best to have your eye doctor check your eyes. Sometimes cataracts produce foggy vision which gradually worsens. Sometimes bright light is painful. You may see bright-colored rings around lights at night. If you want to be reasonably sure you don't develop any of these symptoms, regardless of your age, you should start now to improve your nutrition. A more nutritive diet automatically improves the nutrition of the lens of your eye, which must certainly remove you farther and farther from the danger of cataract.

WHY ARE CATARACTS CALLED THIS PECULIAR NAME?

Cataracts have been known for thousands of years. The ancient Greeks "had a word for it." They thought that a cataract was a flow of cloudy fluid in front of the lens. So they named it just that—a waterfall. We have kept the name, even though we know there is no actual flow of water involved.

Chapter 10

Preventing Cataracts

IT IS IMPOSSIBLE to say categorically that this or that vitamin, mineral, or food is "good for the eyes." The eyes, like other parts of the body, must be nourished by all the various parts of food that make it nutritious. To review, vitamin A is extremely important for good eyesight. A deficiency in vitamin A can cause night blindness, which means that you have difficulty in adjusting to light after darkness, or darkness after light. The B vitamins (especially riboflavin) are also extremely important for healthy eyes. A kind of twilight blindness and a very definite fear of bright light result from not getting enough riboflavin. Vitamin C is important for good eyesight, too, as it is important for every other function of the body. Calcium is needed in the fluids of the eye, and protein is needed to replace eye tissues that have been broken down. And so it goes.

Are any of these important for the prevention of

cataract? All of them are, for they are all necessary to good eye health. You cannot imagine a wonderfully healthy eye, strong, efficient, never giving any trouble, with a cataract beginning to cover the lens! Of course not! What is good for the rest of the eye is also good for the lens. And vice versa.

But we know that certain vitamins may have a somewhat greater importance than others in preventing cataract. For instance, vitamin C is concentrated in the lens of the healthy eyes. Why? We do not know. It is also concentrated in certain tissues in other parts of the body—the adrenal glands, for instance. We cannot help but believe that this concentration of the vitamin must mean that it is needed in that particular spot for some good purpose. Now when we find out that the lens that has a cataract contains very little or no vitamin C, this seems to indicate something very important. Is the lack of vitamin C responsible for the cataract, or is the cataract responsible for the lack of vitamin C? If cataract were a contagious disease spread by germs we would certainly think that the vitamin C had been used up fighting the germs; that's what vitamin C does. But there is no germ involved.

How, then, can we explain this peculiar lack of vitamin C in the lens with a cataract? One function of vitamin C is to keep repairing collagen, the cement between the cells. Could it be that lack of vitamin C has caused these cells to degenerate and form cataracts? It seems likely. And sure enough, we find that researchers have produced cataracts in laboratory

78

animals and then slowed down their growth by giving vitamin C.

Rats fed large amounts of dinitrophenol (the reducing drug that produces animal cataracts, you will remember) responded very rapidly when they were given vitamin C. Other rats developed cataracts when they were fed enormous doses of galactose, a form of sugar. When the vitamin C was given along with the sugar, the appearance of the cataracts was delayed. We have this information from a book called *The Newer Knowledge of Nutrition* by McCollum, Orent-Keiles, and Day (The Macmillan Co., New York, 1944).

RIBOFLAVIN, TOO, IS IMPORTANT FOR EYE HEALTH

We also know that when scurvy (the disease of vitamin C deficiency) is produced in guinea pigs, there is a marked decrease in the vitamin C of the lens. And it is sometimes possible to produce cataracts in guinea pigs on what is called a scorbutic diet, that is, a diet containing little or no vitamin C. The reason this is difficult may be that cataracts result from deficiency in several different vitamins, not just vitamin C. So the guinea pigs whose diet contains plenty of other vitamins may not get cataract.

McCollum and his associates (see above) also tell us that they have a report from a Dr. Josephson indicating that he gave from 15 to 300 milligrams of vitamin C daily to patients with cataracts; marked improvement followed. Within a week, mature cataracts became transparent enough to allow some vision.

Vitamin B$_2$—riboflavin—is extremely important for eye health. The eye is one of the most sensitive organs in the body to a deficiency in riboflavin. In fact, if you are suffering from any peculiar eye symptom, try taking many times the minimum amount of riboflavin each day, no matter what medical treatment you are getting for your eyes. The riboflavin is bound to help. And it's very scarce in most of our diets, so there's a good chance that you may be short.

In one experiment, rats kept on a diet containing no riboflavin got cataracts—almost 100 per cent of them! It occurred only in rats who were deprived of the vitamin at an early age, not those who got the deficient diet after they were mature. Could it be that the very widespread incidence of cataracts today is the direct result of lack of riboflavin in the diet of folks who were growing up 50, 60, or 70 years ago? In other experiments such clear-cut results have not been achieved. It is believed that possibly these laboratory diets were not as deficient in riboflavin as the investigators thought. However, nutrition books in general relate deficiency in riboflavin with cataract.

Could then the reason for cataracts in newborn babies be lack of riboflavin and vitamin C in the mother's diet? There seems to be no reason why not. The mineral calcium is also related to the formation of cataract. Cantarow, in his book *Calcium Metabolism and Calcium Therapy* (Lea and Febiger, 1931), says that a lack of calcium in the diet allows the cataract to form. He also says that calcium seems to be necessary for the body to use vitamin C correctly. Remember what we said about not just one but many, many elements being important for any body function?

Finally we have abundant evidence that a diet low in protein is likely to make one susceptible to cataracts. Researchers have been able to produce cataracts in animals by feeding them diets in which one or another of the important amino acids (forms of protein) is lacking. The essential amino acids work together—one cannot function without all of them. Adding the missing amino acids to the diet delayed the appearance of the cataracts.

TREATING INCIPIENT CATARACT WITH DIET

Now read to what one practicing doctor has to say about preventing and treating cataracts, for this gentleman has been doing wonderful work among cataract patients. Dr. Donald T. Atkinson, of San Antonio, Texas, wrote in the February, 1952, issue of *The Eye, Ear, Nose, and Throat Monthly* an article entitled "Malnutrition as an Ethiological [causative] Factor in Senile Cataract."

He tells us first that there has been a lot of discussion about the possibility of cataract resulting from dehydration of the lens; that is, perhaps the water has been extracted from it. Cholera patients, it seems, go blind in the last stages of their illness because the

81

lenses of their eyes dry out. A frog placed in salt water soon develops cataract because the salt extracts the water from the lens of the eye. Put the frog back into fresh water and the cataract disappears. Dr. Atkinson does not mention the danger of too much salt in the diet of human beings, but his story about the frog makes us wonder whether the vast amount of oversalting we do has anything to do with cataract.

Dr. Atkinson became intensely interested in the relationship of diet to cataract when he was treating the wife of a young physician for cataract. At about the same time, he says, there were numerous other cases of cataract among young people in that part of the country. He remarked to himself that all these young people seemed to be remarkably badly nourished, including the physician's wife.

All of them lived mainly on corn products and salt pork. Their principal beverage was coffee; they drank little water. Fresh foods were almost nonexistent in their diets. As for bread, they ate refined wheat and corn bread raised with bicarbonate of soda—not yeast. The soda rapidly destroyed whatever vitamins might have remained in their bread. And the lack of yeast removed the one last source of B vitamins that might have remained to them.

So Dr. Atkinson began to suggest to his patients who were just beginning to get cataracts that they adopt diets rich in some of the vitamins, especially vitamin C—cabbage, oranges, carrots, tomatoes, rutabagas, turnips, and so on. Result? Several patients who really followed the diet found that their cata-

82

racts were getting no bigger; in some cases they improved.

The other food factor that Dr. Atkinson used in treating his cataract patients was chlorophyll. He reminds us that green plants are more nutritious than dried ones; animals do better on green pasture than dried hay, as evidenced by their half-starved look in early spring and the rapidity with which they recover once they begin to eat green grass again. The chemical properties of chlorophyll, the green coloring matter of plants, are almost the same as the properties of hemoglobin, the red coloring matter in the blood. The chemical formula differs only in the fact that an atom of iron in the hemoglobin molecule corresponds to the atom of magnesium in the chlorophyll.

"It is a very engrossing fact," he says, "as it now appears, in the retardation of cataract that the formula of chlorophyll and hemoglobin are so nearly alike. Willstatter found carotin, a type of chlorophyll in the body of fresh carrots, and he suspected that its administration had a wholesome effect on vision. So far as I know I was the first to prescribe a diet of green tops of garden vegetables to cataract patients and I still find that this diet has its advantages in incipient cataract cases."

WILL NOT SUCH A DIET PREVENT CATARACT?

This is the kind of diet Dr. Atkinson uses in cases of cataracts: a greatly increased intake of water—from 8 to 10 glasses a day in addition to the tea, coffee, and whatever other beverages the patient is drinking. From a list of the green tops of 6 selected garden vegetables he has them add one as "greens" to the diet daily. We suppose they can choose whichever they like best. Then, in addition, he gives them chlorophyll tablets and large doses of vitamin C (as much as 1,000 milligrams a day). He also gives them 200,000 units of vitamin A every day. Finally, each patient is required to have a pint of milk and two eggs daily. (Look over this diet if you are worried about cataract and see whether your daily diet is as good.)

At the time he wrote this article (1952), Dr. Atkinson had 450 patients with elementary cataract. Over a period of 11 years a number of these cataracts had not worsened. Formerly his patients went through the regular routine with a cataract, letting it mature and then having an operation. Now, he says, only a limited number have had to have operations.

We think we know another reason for the success of Dr. Atkinson's diet, quite apart from the amount of chlorophyll in it: it contains plenty of vitamins A and C. The greens from the garden are rich in vitamins A and C as well as riboflavin—the B vitamin we found in our research to be important for the prevention of cataract. There is calcium, too, in those green leafy

84

vegetables—lots of it. Then, too, when one is eating plenty of fresh vegetables and fruits, he just can't dilute his diet with a lot of white bread and rich desserts. He just hasn't the room. And this is bound to be helpful, too.

We would add to Dr. Atkinson's diet for preventing cataract brewer's yeast, which is the richest possible source of riboflavin and all the other B vitamins. We would certainly add bone meal for additional calcium and other naturally occurring minerals. And we would add vitamin E, to preserve the health of blood vessels, thus assuring better nutrition for all the tissues of the body.

A JUDGE'S EXPERIENCE

Many years ago I read of an experience of a judge who had gotten cataracts from sitting on his judge's bench for many years facing the glare of a large window. He sued the state but lost his case (on what grounds I cannot remember). It is a good reminder that while working at a desk or reading, one should sit so that the light comes in from the side.

Chapter 11

Rutin for Eye Disorders

RUTIN, ONE COMPONENT of vitamin P, was once administered to a group of patients with glaucoma, the tragic eye disease in which the pressure inside the eyeball rises. Among 26 patients who received 20 milligrams of rutin three times a day, 17 noticed a fall in the pressure inside the eye, in four the results were not definite, and five subjects noticed no change.

We found an extremely interesting article by L. B. Somerville-Large on the use of rutin in ophthalmology in the *Transactions of the Ophthalmological Society of the United Kingdom* (Vol. 69, pages 615-617, 1949-1950). Dr. Somerville-Large states that "in the eye we have what appears to be the only opportunity the human body affords of actually observing lesions [disorders] associated with capillary dysfunction. We must, therefore, forgive our medical colleagues for their caution in recognizing the value of rutin." He goes on to tell us that the tiny blood vessels in the eye can be studied by the ophthalmologist. It is actually the only place in the body where blood vessels can be directly observed. These tiny capillaries in the eye are packed closely together, and they have a wider "bore" than other capillaries in the body.

He says that the commonest conditions in which the capillaries seem to be out of order are diabetes, toxic and inflammatory conditions, high blood pressure, and hardening of the arteries. Hypertension (high blood pressure) of itself has no relation to capillary fragility, he says, 6 to 10 per cent of those hypertension sufferers who do have increased capillary fragility also suffer from hemorrhages in the retina of the eye and cerebral or brain hemorrhages. He gives doses of two 60-milligram tablets of rutin three times a day, making a total dosage of 360 milligrams daily. "I find," says he, "that the larger doses give a more rapid and more complete negative result to capillary fragility tests." Incidentally, he always combines the rutin with 200 milligrams of vitamin C daily.

It is interesting to note that throughout the discussion of vitamin P and rutin in medical literature, it is suggested that vitamin P and vitamin C work closely together and better results are always obtained when they are used together. Note, too, that Dr. Somerville-Large gives quite a large dose of vitamin C— 200 milligrams. At the present time the official recommendation for the minimum daily intake of vitamin C is only 70 milligrams, and it is believed that most of us don't even get that much! Does it not seem reasonable that two or three times this amount of vitamin C every day might do a lot to prevent the capillary fragility which is responsible for so much distress today? Remember that vitamin C is also involved in keeping the intercellular membranes healthy.

In conclusion, Dr. Somerville-Large states that in his experience he has not yet "met a case in which the capillary fragility skin test has not been reduced with rutin to well within normal limits." In speaking of the length of time it is necessary to continue taking the rutin, he says, "To me at the present time it looks like a life sentence. Whenever rutin has been discontinued the capillary fragility has again increased. Also, if the rutin is discontinued and the vitamin C alone persisted with, again the capillary fragility increases."

One last example of the use of rutin is treating capillary fragility: Bicknell and Prescott, in *Vitamins in Medicine*, tell of 12 children in a group of 100 allergic children who were treated with 100 to 150 milligrams of vitamin P daily for six months. At the end of this time their capillary resistance became normal.

HOW MUCH VITAMIN P ARE YOU GETTING IN EVERYDAY MEALS?

What application can we make of all these experiences to our daily life? First of all, if vitamin P (of which rutin is a part) is really a vitamin, how much of it do we need every day? The Federation of the American Societies for Experimental Biology have voted to discontinue the use of the term "vitamin" in relation to vitamin P. They decided that it has not been proved as yet that these substances (the flavones) are essential to good health and that their absence in diet will cause any disorder that can be cured by administering them. However, it is interesting to note that people in other countries, and in this country as well, go right on calling the flavones "vitamin P." Bicknell and Prescott state that the daily requirement may be not less than 33 units daily "and possibly considerably more."

Just like vitamin C, vitamin P is destroyed by cooking in an open vessel; so much of the vitamin P value of food is lost in cooking. Once again we are faced with the absolute necessity for eating plenty of fresh raw fruits and vegetables, for it is in these that vitamin P is found in the largest amounts, along with vitamin C.

The rutin concentrate used by doctors in treating hypertensive patients is made from buckwheat. Rutin occurs chiefly in the buckwheat leaves, which may contain as much as 7 or 8 per cent rutin. It is rapidly destroyed when the leaves are dried slowly, so they must be processed with the greatest care. After the leaves are completely dried, there seems to be no further loss of rutin.

If you are suffering from high blood pressure and your doctor advises taking rutin to avoid any possibility of a stroke, we would certainly go along with his advice on the basis of the evidence we have collected. If you are perfectly healthy and interested in preserving the state of your blood vessels so you will not suffer from these disorders later, then by all means see that you get, every day, plenty of the foods in which vitamin P (and hence rutin) occurs, along with vitamin C. Of course, you should always get enough vitamin C, for it is thought to be one of the most essential food elements for good health. Now it appears that vitamin P, always associated with vitamin C in foods, may be of great value as well.

Here is a list of foods that are rich in vitamin P, with their vitamin C content as well. Notice that just as rose hips are many, many times richer in vitamin C than any other food, so too they are especially rich in vitamin P.

	Vitamin P Content, Units	*Vitamin C Content, Milligrams*
Apricots	75-100 in 8 apricots	4
Blackberry	60-100 in ¾ cup	3
Black currant	200-500 in 1 cup	150
Cabbage (summer)	100 in 1 cup, raw	50
Cherry, black	60-100 in 12 large cherries	12
Grape, black	500-1,000 in 1 small bunch	3
Grape, white	500-1,000 in 1 small bunch	4
Parsley	130 in 1 cup	70
Plum	50-200 in 3 medium plums	5
Prune	300-400 in 8 medium prunes	4
Rose hips	240-680 in 100 grams	500 to 6,000

Chapter 12

Contact Lenses

CONTACT LENSES ENDANGER THE EYES

WHEN THE IDEA OF contact lenses first originated, the reasons for using them were much clearer than they are today. Movie stars and athletes were the chief consumers, and their need was obvious. The style of glasses, until 10 or 15 years ago, was far from flattering. They were either encased in round solid gold or silver metal frames, or they were rimless and angular. Glasses were anything but attractive, and for anyone whose livelihood depended upon pleasing appearance, contact lenses seemed to be an answer to a prayer. The glasses in those days were fragile, too. If they were dropped, they were gone, so athletes were faced with a real problem in trying to keep them from being broken in a game. Contact lenses would at least be a practical consideration here.

What about the situation today? The shapes of the

new frames, and materials used in them, have made eyeglasses a fashion focus for the ladies. It is the style now to call attention to eyeglasses by studding them with rhinestones, shaping them exotically and coloring them to match any ensemble. Some women with good vision are actually envious because they can't take advantage of the fashion values of cleverly designed spectacle frames.

Not only are the frames beautiful but they are made so that the lenses can take a lot of punishment. The plastic frames have a valuable resilience, so that the shock of being dropped is lessened; and because they can be set deep in a plastic frame, the lens surface is not likely to be scratched or cracked when they are dropped. Actually, the original reasons for the development of contact lenses have just about disappeared, yet they are more sought after than ever before. Over 6 million Americans wear contact lenses, and the number is increasing by 500,000 a year. It's a $200,000,000 business. If all these contact lenses are being used, why do we disagree with the thousands of doctors who recommend and prescribe them? We do not believe contact lenses are safe.

THEY CAN LEAD TO SERIOUS IMPAIRMENT OF VISION

One eye specialist after the other has expressed caution or true fear at the prospect of prescribing contact lenses. In the *New York Times* (June 2, 1960), the House of Delegates of the American Medical Association was quoted as saying, ". . . the use of such lenses [i.e., contact] is not entirely without hazard . . . [and] this House views with grave concern the use of contact lenses." Said Dr. R. O. Rychner, ophthalmologist of the National Medical Foundation for Eye Care in New York, "The use of contact lenses can at times lead to serious permanent impairment of vision."

How true that statement is can be gathered from what an AMA (American Medical Association) meeting in Miami was told by Capt. R. K. Lanshe, an eye specialist serving with the Marine Corps: corneal strangulation can result from wearing contact lenses with too sharp an inner curvature. This lens curve creates a suction-cup effect that can prevent the metabolic exchanges of gases, hypertonic tears, and heat.

The U. S. *Armed Forces Medical Journal* is quoted in *Newsweek* (August 8, 1960) as warning of "potential danger of eye infection and of injury" from wearing contact lenses. *Good Housekeeping* magazine (June, 1960) tells of five leading ophthalmologists who observed cases where corneal damage resulted. One specialist in lens, fitting said, "Corneal abrasions are not uncommon. Though they heal quickly in most cases, you can get scarring and reduced vision. I tell all my patients that there is danger in wearing contact lenses." A routine sampling of 16 ophthalmologists across the United States brought out some startling facts: 15 of them had treated corneal injuries resulting from contact lenses, and 4 out of these had

93

handled cases in which the eye was lost as a result of the damage.

TROUBLE AND EXPENSE

The whole contact lens procedure is so much trouble and expense, aside from the real danger always present to the eye, that one wonders why anyone has the patience to bother with them. The price is prohibitive: it averages about $200 a pair. But perhaps the words of a contact lens purchaser who told of his experiences in a letter to *Consumer Bulletin* (January, 1960) would be of greater persuasion than our opinion. He says, "At a contact lens specialist, I bought a pair of contact lenses. The standard price is, or was, $180.00. This, in my case included a pair of reading glasses to be worn with them and a bottle of liquid, which I was directed to use every time I used them. Because of the ever-present danger of losing the lenses by misplacement or having them fall out of the eye, I was advised to buy an insurance policy. Annual premium $15.00. . . . I could see quite well with the lenses. There the satisfaction ended. Putting them in the eye requires the use of a special fluid, considerable skill and practice, a mirror and, preferably, privacy. . . . Taking them out is another trick. . . . This I know: Any talk about 'throwing away' your glasses is pure deception. You will need them.

"Having thought contact lenses primarily suited to outdoor activities, on boats (or swimming), my experience of losing them is just another time I was played for a sucker and should have known better. Nothing could be what the ads say contact lenses are. Fortunately, the financial loss was not serious for me, but I do regret the evenings I spent with the cussed things in my eyes, crying copiously, looking down only, night after night."

That's one man's misery, but his feelings are not unusual. The discomfort and precautions involved in getting used to and wearing contact lenses are monumental, even for those who are said to have made the adjustment with relative ease. As a rule, the wearer suffers stinging, burning, and the sensation of a foreign body in the eye at first, and these annoyances often last for several weeks. No wonder. The lens is a thin plastic disc a little smaller than a dime, and it rests directly on the cornea, separated only by a film of tears which holds the lens in place. The wearer always feels as though there is something in his eye, and indeed there is: something as big as a dime in an organ sensitive enough that even a tiny speck of dust is enough to cause discomfort!

One person tells of a visit to his ophthalmologist, who had just finished with a patient using contact lenses. The doctor told him that the previous patient was unable to endure wearing contact lenses for more than one hour. When the man suggested sunflower seeds to help strengthen the eyes against the irritation of the contact lenses, the doctor was skeptical but decided to give it a try. The patient, after using the sunflower seeds for a short time, reported that the contact lenses could be worn for three hours without removal, and attributed the improvement solely to the sunflower seeds. If you know someone who is suffering similarly, perhaps your suggestion that he do the same would save him much discomfort.

And do you think anyone could possibly remember all the restrictions concerning contact lenses? Here are some from *Scope* (July 3, 1960):

"Patients must be warned never to experiment with the lens, nor engage in competition for length of wearing time with other patients.

"They must not build up the wearing time too rapidly or irregularly, nor wear the lenses for irregular periods from day to day or while sleeping. The lens should be removed when conjunctivitis (inflammation of the eye-covering membrane), blepharitis (inflammation of the eyelid itself) or upper respiratory infections are present. Strict personal habits of hygiene must be followed (using saliva for cleaning the lenses is unthinkable), and gentle insertion and removal of the lens is absolutely necessary."

The *Good Housekeeping* article mentioned above adds these dissuaders: Certain people should never even try to wear contact lenses—diabetics; those with chronic colds or sinusitis; extra dry, teary, or abnormally protruding eyes. And those who do wear them must constantly be on the alert against lenses roughened in use; against dust, dirt, nicotine on the lenses; against rubbing the eyes; or against wearing lenses while eyes are irritated by colds, hay fever, or sties. Any one of these can cause a scratch on the cornea, which can lead to serious eye infection. Any break in the surface of the cornea gives germs a chance to enter, multiply, and cause infection. These can cause corneal scars that may reduce vision; worse, an ulcer may develop which, in some extensive cases, requires the eye's removal.

That's the story on contact lenses. How anyone who is seriously interested in the health of his eyes could even consider using them is something we cannot understand.

Chapter 13

Aniseikonia, a Recently Discovered Eye Disorder

A FRIEND OF OURS had headaches for 20 years—blinding, searing, nauseating headaches that put her to bed at least three or four days out of every month. She had taken 30 or 40 different treatments, all to no avail. Her glasses (for astigmatism) were changed regularly, and each time her glasses were changed her headaches grew worse. Her friends began to believe that the headaches must be a sign of neurosis. She herself was at the point of complete desperation and I had made arrangements to have an examination for brain tumor.

A neighbor who was an optometrist asked if she would stop in at his office before she went out of town for her examination. Figuring that she had nothing to lose, she did. With a series of curious and very complicated machines, Dr. Benton Freeman of Allentown, Pa., tested her eyes and told her she had aniseikonia, a maladjustment of eyesight. Over a period of six months he adjusted and readjusted a set of curved lenses. When they were perfectly adjusted for the degree of aniseikonia that she had, he made permanent lenses for her. This all took place five years ago. From the time the first aniseikonic lens was placed in the frame of her glasses, she has not had a headache. What is perhaps even more surprising, she continually bit her fingernails down to the quick during the years when she had headaches. A month after the headaches stopped, she found to her amazement that she had stopped biting her nails.

Aniseikonia is an eye disorder in which each eye sees objects at a different distance and different position in space. The constant effort made by her brain to adjust these two images was the cause of our friend's headaches. The aniseikonic lenses cannot cure this maladjustment of her eyes, but so long as she wears them she is free from all symptoms. In her case, each time her lenses were adjusted for astigmatism, her aniseikonia became worse, because then she saw each of the two images even more clearly.

Aniseikonia was discovered at Dartmouth a number of years ago, and research and experimentation were done on a grant from John D. Rockefeller, whose own headaches were cured by aniseikonic lenses. It is estimated that more than 1 per cent of our population may have aniseikonia. There are only about 25 doctors in the country who have the equipment to test for it. They can tell you in a half hour whether you have aniseikonia or not and if you have they can, without fail, prescribe lenses to correct it.

It is a lengthy procedure, but certainly well worth the time and money.

Dr. Freeman had patients from all over the Eastern United States. Some of them were brought to his office in an ambulance, if they had broken their lenses, because their symptoms were so violent without their glasses. Many ophthalmologists refuse to believe in the existence of such a disorder, even after they have interviewed these same patients, some of whom cannot stand on their feet or sit in a chair without falling once they take off their glasses. If you believe aniseikonia may be causing your headaches, we'd suggest that you write to Dartmouth and ask for the name of the doctor nearest to you who can test you for it. Address Dr. Robert E. Bannon, Dartmouth Eye Institute, Hanover, New Hampshire 03755.

Chapter 14

The Bates System of Eye Training

NOT SO LONG AGO a new system for training eye-sight which would make glasses unnecessary became popular. Later, enthusiasm died down considerably, and we have not seen anything about the "Bates method" for quite a long time. We feel the time is ripe to revive interest in this very sensible and successful method of treating eyes and preventing eye disorders.

Dr. W. H. Bates, a New York oculist, concluded that the great majority of visual defects are functional and due to faulty habits of eye use. These habits develop from strain and tension. By teaching his patients how to relax and how to use their eyes in a relaxed way, Dr. Bates found that vision was improved and that errors in their sight were corrected.

Actually, when you stop to think of it, why should any of us be content to wear glasses? If the defect were in the knee instead, would we be as content to go on a crutch? Of course not! We would try every doctor and every known technique that might bring our knee back to usefulness so that we could discard the crutch. But we seem to take it for granted that eventually, if not at once, we will have to be fitted with glasses. We also grant that thereafter we will always have to wear them, while our eyes (depending on the glasses as our legs would on a crutch) get progressively worse, needing stronger glasses from time to time.

On the other hand, if we did not use our legs correctly, we would probably need a crutch in time. And so with our eyes. At any rate, this is the basis of Dr. Bates' theory, which is explained in his own book, *Better Eyesight Without Glasses* (Holt, Rinehart and Winston, New York, 1943), and another book, *The Art of Seeing* (Harper & Row, New York, 1942), written by the famous English author, Aldous Huxley. Mr. Huxley, who very nearly lost his sight at the age of sixteen, attributes to the Bates system his recovery of sight in one eye and a great improvement of sight in the other.

According to Mr. Huxley, ophthalmologists are interested in the physiological aspects of seeing. Artificial lenses in spectacles work mechanically to correct physiological sight defects. But what of the mental, the psychological, aspect of vision? Isn't it possible that by learning to use the eyes correctly one may correct defects that have probably been caused by using the eyes incorrectly?

102

In his book Mr. Huxley describes many of the Bates exercises. We have room for only a few here. Perhaps the most important is "palming," whose purpose is to relax the eyes. Bates students are requested to "palm" often. Resting the elbows on a table, cover the eyes with the hands, one hand to each eye. Rest the palm of the hand on the cheek, the fingers on the forehead so that the hand does not touch the eye itself. You should see nothing but black. If there are spots, flashes of light or other disturbances, keep palming, relaxed and effortless, until you see nothing but black. It will help to think of the color black or to think of some pleasant happening in the past, "seeing" the incident in your mind's eye, with your physical eyes closed.

A second helpful exercise from the Bates method is blinking. According to Mr. Huxley, one outstanding symptom of the person with poor eyesight is his tendency to stare. He is so eager to see well, he wants so desperately not to miss a thing, he knows his eyes are bad, and so he makes a great effort and strains hard to see better. All that he actually does is to make himself see worse.

"Movement," says Mr. Huxley, ". . . is one of the indispensable conditions of sensing and perceiving. But so long as the eyelids are kept tense and relatively immobile, the eyes themselves will remain tense and relatively immobile. Hence anyone who wishes to acquire the art of seeing well must cultivate the habit of frequent and effortless blinking. . . ."

103

He suggests a "blinking drill" every hour or so, followed by a few seconds of relaxing the eyes by closing them. Half a dozen light butterfly-blinks, then closing, another half-dozen blinks, then closing, and so on for about a minute. This kind of exercise is especially important for those engaged in close work, where the eyes can be harmed by straining and staring.

SOME EYE EXERCISES THAT ARE FUN TO TRY

Another good habit is to squeeze the eyes shut every so often—wrinkling up all the other face muscles at the same time. Do this when you are tempted to rub your eyes, for you should never, never rub your eyes for any reason at all. Nor should you massage them, but you can rub the temples, which will relax and soothe the eyes, and you can rub and knead the muscles in the upper part of the nape of the neck, which will help.

"Flashing" is another exercise recommended in the Bates method—an important one for making the eye more mobile and increasing those powers of the mind that perceive and interpret what one sees. Flashing is the opposite of staring. Rather than straining to see all parts of an object, glance at it quickly, almost casually and then close your eyes and remember what the object looked like. You will be surprised to find that your physical eye "saw" more than you knew it saw. With your eyes closed, you will be able to remember far more about the object than you were conscious of seeing.

Children who are re-learning how to use their eyes have no trouble with "flashing," for they are much less self-conscious than adults. "A child is shown some object, say a domino, or a printed letter or word, from a distance at which he cannot normally see. He is told to take a flashing glance at it, then close his eyes and 'reach up into the air for it.' The child obeys the order quite literally, raises a hand, closes it on emptiness, then lowers it, opens it, looks into his palm and gives the correct answer, as though he were reading from notes."

"Shifting" is another valuable exercise, as Mr. Huxley says: "People with normal vision keep their eyes and attention shifting unconsciously in a series of almost imperceptible small movements from point to point. People with defective vision, on the contrary, greatly reduce the number of such movements and tend to stare. It is, therefore, necessary for them to build up consciously the habit of small-scale shifting which they acquired unconsciously in childhood and subsequently lost."

When you are "shifting" you don't try to see the whole thing at which you are looking. Make yourself look at it piece by piece, studying first this portion, then that. If it is as large a thing as a house, look first at the windows, then at the roof, then at the door, and so on. If it is as small as a printed letter M, look first at the straight line, then at the slanting down line, then at the line that slants up, and finally at the last upright line. In this way your eye, instead of staring at the letter, will move over it, bit by bit. This is good training for good sight.

IMAGINATION IS IMPORTANT IN EYE EXERCISES

One very amusing exercise which apparently Mr. Huxley often uses is "nose writing." Sit comfortably in an easy chair and imagine you have a pencil attached to the end of your nose. In fact, everything you do in this exercise involves your imagination. Using the imaginary pencil attached to your nose, begin to write, moving your shoulders and head as you need to. Imagine that you are drawing a large circle. If it looks uneven to your "inner eye," draw over and over it until you have a fairly presentable circle. Then draw a line through the center, another at right angles to it, and so on. The object of this exercise is to relax and rest the eyes. Of course you must use your imagination in a lively fashion throughout. And this, too, teaches you how to use your imagination; you will need it later on in some of the more difficult eye exercises which according to Dr. Bates, will improve your eyesight greatly.

It is impossible to sum up in a sentence the full meaning of the Bates exercises. But it is, generally speaking, a treatment designed to correct eyesight by teaching the individual to use his eyes correctly. This means that he will see correctly.

Dr. Bates book describes some astonishing cures of

eye disorders all the way from myopia to glaucoma. He tells of cases among his own patients where the prescribed treatment (without glasses) brought relief from pains of neuralgia, headaches, and other physical symptoms, aside from cases of improvement in actual vision that sound almost unbelievable. During his lifetime Dr. Bates suffered from the persecution that is universally visited upon those who discover something new in the way of treatment and use it successfully. He was called quack and charlatan. "It is quite true," says Mr. Huxley, "that oculists and optometrists have never observed such phenomena as are described by Bates and his followers. But this is because they have never had any dealings with patients who had learned to use their organs of vision in a relaxed, unrestrained way."

We would suggest that you get Dr. Bates book out of your local library. If they do not have it, perhaps they will order it for you.

SAILORS' EYESIGHT

According to the evidence, sailors usually have very good eyesight. This could come from the same principle as the Bates method of eye exercises. Aboard ship, hundreds of times a day, they shift their focus from near points on the ship to the distant horizon. Their eyes move constantly.

Chapter 15

Therapy for Crossed Eyes

A PERSON WITH CROSSED EYES sees two objects when he's looking at one, because each eye views the same object from a widely different angle. He squints or tilts his head, unconsciously trying to combine the two images or ignore one of them. Neither attempt fully succeeds. Eventually such a strabismus victim stops trying to see with both eyes. When he looks at things with only one eye, he sees only one image. Using one eye becomes a convenient habit, and soon the other eye becomes incapable of focusing on anything. Functionally, it is blind.

The basic cause of crossed eyes is the unequal pull of eye muscles. If the muscle on one side of the eye pulls harder than the muscle on the other side, the eye "looks" toward the side with the stronger muscle. An eye doctor works to equalize the pull of the muscles until the eye in repose is directed straight ahead. Sometimes glasses alone can force better direction, but rarely.

Another familiar device used to treat crossed eyes is an eye patch. The stronger eye is covered, forcing the weaker one to do all the sight work. The confusion of the double image is immediately resolved, and the idea is that increased work will restore muscular control of the weaker eye. Unfortunately, once the patch is removed the eye usually goes right back to the old position.

Failure with these measures used to leave surgery as the last resort. The surgeon shortens the weaker eye muscle and equalizes the pull on both sides of the eye to make it look straight ahead. Sometimes several operations are required before the proper alignment is achieved.

SURGERY UNSATISFACTORY

Sometimes eyes apparently respond to the operation but still lack the versatility necessary for good vision. Peripheral vision may be obscured; distant focus might be fine, but not closeup; the ability to follow moving objects or adjust focus rapidly from near to far away just isn't there.

Doctors would junk surgery as a treatment for crossed eyes if they could. The results are so unpredictable that one successful operation out of four is considered a pretty good average. In a child born with strabismus, chances are even less that surgery will get the two eyes to work together perfectly. A good result depends largely on a very early operation; some patients are no more than 18 months old. As many as 50 children a year die during operations

109

to straighten crossed eyes. The recognized uncertainty and risks of surgery are so great that conservative Johns Hopkins University Hospital has established an Orthoptic Center that concentrates on treatments other than surgery for correcting eye problems.

Important among these treatments is exercise therapy, a technique deserving wider knowledge and application than it has yet received. Exercise therapy is simple, safe, and, according to Dr. William M. Ludlam, of New York City, successful in about 70 per cent of the cases. The clincher: in most cases, even persons who have surgery need eye exercises later to round out the results. Parents are certainly sensible to try the exercises first.

The child in visual training works at machines that stimulate a variety of visual situations and help him adjust his sight to them. He repeats sighting patterns that force his eyes into proper positioning and coordination. Eventually the eyes can do the work with minimal assistance from glasses—sometimes without glasses.

The theory of eye exercise for improved vision is not a new one. The Bates system, evolved several generations ago, and described in Chapter 14 prescribed general exercises for eye strengthening and more specific ones for individual eye disabilities. Modern visual training has greatly refined the approaches and predictability of eye exercise. New equipment makes exercising easier and helps to maintain interest long enough to get results.

110

PRENATAL DIET IMPORTANT

Most physicians agree that a tendency toward visual problems is inborn. This means that prenatal care can have some influence in preventing weaknesses. Throughout the pregnancy, a healthful diet, high in protein and other vitamin-rich foods will help to ensure strong muscle tissue and healthful nerves that will work toward proper eye control in the expected baby.

When eye trouble is already present, researchers have found that some specific nutrients can minimize the damage. In *Presse Medicale* (April 25, 1959) two Parisian physicians reported that vitamin E helps in treating nearsighted youngsters. During 10 years of research they stopped deterioration and even improved vision with the vitamin. A check on these patients after 8 years showed that the effects are lasting.

The treatment calls for one or two 50-milligram tablets of vitamin E first thing in the morning every day for three months. After this three-month treatment, a lapse of several weeks is allowed; then another three-month series is given. Drs. C. and G. Desusclade believe this stabilizes the improvement. They suggest that the treatment be repeated every year while the child is growing up.

Vitamin E-rich foods include beans, beef liver, eggs, green peas, sweet potatoes, and salad oils. All seed foods, including sunflower and pumpkin, contain vitamin E. To be sure your family gets as much

111

vitamin E as necessary, add wheat germ oil or vitamin E capsules to the other food supplements they take.

Dr. P. A. Gardner reported improvement in myopic children who are given increased amounts of animal protein in their diet. *Food Field Reporter* (April 27, 1959) said that two groups of children, all nearsighted, participated in an experiment in which one group got increased amounts of animal protein and the second ate an ordinary diet. The untreated children in the five to seven age group showed a visual deterioration four times greater than the children getting a high protein diet. In the eight to nine year group, deterioration in the group without extra protein in the diet was three times greater. In children twelve or over, actual improvement in nearsightedness occurred in those taking the largest quantities of animal protein.

If for no other reason than to protect your children's eyes, protein foods deserve a prominent place in your family's daily menu. Meat, fish, eggs, and other high protein foods should appear at least once a day, more if possible.

It is unfortunately true that surgery is the last resort in some eye problems. Sometimes nothing but very strong glasses will do just to keep the eyes from getting worse. But for most people with functional eye problems, visual training can be a ticket to good vision. For all of us, good nutrition is good insurance against eye trouble.

Chapter 16

Various Things

NEARSIGHTEDNESS

MOST NEAR-SIGHTED PEOPLE, we imagine, feel that any hazards connected with their eye condition are remedied by the proper glasses. But an article in *Industrial Medicine and Surgery* for October, 1951, tells us that they run a risk of permanently injuring their eyes or even going blind if they engage in work that involves heavy lifting, straining, or possible bumps on the head.

Dr. Hedwig S. Kuhn, author of the article, says that an extremely near-sighted person suffers attendant stretching of the eyeball and various changes in the retina of the eye. These, in heavy lifting or with a sudden bump of the head, can cause a detachment of the retina. Usually the person is unaware that anything has happened to his eye, and the condition may go on untended for several days, during which time the retina is deprived of its blood supply. Generally, says Dr. Kuhn, this situation results in total loss of vision in the affected eye.

Kuhn's article was written to caution physicians examining job applicants to watch for near-sighted applicants and to make certain they are placed in jobs that do not require heavy lifting, excessive stooping, or the risk of bumps on the head. So if you are very nearsighted, avoid this kind of job and make sure that you don't lift heavy objects around home. Furthermore, now is the time to put white paint over that low-hanging rafter in the cellar or that low ceiling on the attic stairway so that in the future you'll remember to duck and not bump your head.

OVERUSE OF EYES

From the *British Medical Journal* for August 15, 1953, comes a comment on eye damage, made by Dr. J. H. Doggart. Says he, "It is almost impossible to damage the eyes by long hours of reading and sewing, even if great fatigue is experienced at the time."

It has always seemed to us that using your eyes is good for them; especially if you use your eyes properly in the relaxed fashion as Dr. Bates taught in his books on the subject, you can use them just about indefinitely without doing them harm.

AGING EYESIGHT

Dr. Nathan W. Shock *Newsweek* (October 2, 1950) reports that after age fifty, nearly everyone suffers eye changes which interfere with good vision. At sixty there is a definite drop in color discrimination.

Dr. Hobson points out that the lens of the eye is a very sensitive index to age. It seems that among otherwise healthy people, the ability of the eye lens to accommodate falls steadily until the age of fifty, when it remains stationary. "We can say," he goes on, "with a fair degree of accuracy, that in the great majority of people, physiological senescence in the human lens is reached at the age of fifty, but it begins at quite an early age—even before puberty."

In other words, the ability of the eye to see at long distances or to adjust itself immediately to seeing things that are quite close is actually at its lowest ebb at the age of fifty, or thereabouts. It doesn't get much worse from then on. The inability of the lens of the eye to adjust to close work is, of course, the reason most of us wear reading glasses or bifocals after middle age. It is interesting to know that this degeneration of the eye lens begins during adolescence and progresses quite steadily until the age of 50—and apparently does not get much worse from then on. So if you have managed to do without reading glasses up to the age of 50, perhaps you will be able to do without them completely!

Dr. Hobson tells us that both visual accuracy and how quickly you see things are affected by age. The amount of light you need becomes increasingly important, too. These changes can be detected by the age of twenty!

SUNGLASSES

It may sound silly to warn people not to wear sunglasses indoors, but strange as it seems, some people do. According to the *Science News Letter* for August 11, 1956, the eyes become used to a low level of light when we wear dark glasses outdoors. Inside, however, we need all the light there is. And if we are going to spend an equal amount of time indoors and out, the only wise precaution is to remove dark glasses when we come into the shade or the house. Remember, sunflower seeds are a natural for eye health!

While on the subject, I should say that I too used to wear sunglasses at the beach. But now that I eat sunflower seeds, I can stand the glare of the sun there.

I believe also that if people were to eat sunflower seeds regularly they would not have to wear sunglasses on ordinary city streets.

TELEVISION

Television seems to present little risk to eyesight if certain precautions are observed.

Each new invention of technological skill seems to be accompanied by its own hazards. In some cases these are confined to a special group, depending on the kind of work done, the food eaten, the medicine taken, and so forth. But there are some recent inventions whose well-nigh universal use makes them potential hazards for us all. Most American homes have television these days—or at any rate most American families spend some time every week watching television. Naturally, parents are concerned over the possible eye damage that may result in enthusiastic young followers of cowboy serials, baseball games, and children's programs.

A booklet by Dr. Benjamin Rones, "Does Television Damage the Eyes?" has been published by the National Society for the Prevention of Blindness. The booklet is devoted to explaining "how we can make the best use of our eyes in viewing television and how to avoid possible discomfort."

CLEAR IMAGE IS VITAL

How important is the clearness with which the image is seen? Of primary importance, says Dr. Rones. In or near large cities, where reception from local stations is good, a clear-cut image on the screen is easy to obtain. But just as many television sets are in use in distant areas where faulty reception cannot provide a clear-cut picture. The flickering of the picture is bound to result in headaches and eye fatigue. If your room is small, increasing the size of the screen does no good, for it only blows up all the imperfections of the picture and gives your eyes even more distress. If your television room is large, so that you can sit quite far away from the screen, the imperfections are minimized by a larger screen.

LIGHTING THE TELEVISION ROOM

Most people realize that turning off all the lights in the room is a mistake, for the lighting of the room should not provide too great a contrast to the light from the screen. Shifting one's eyes back and forth from the brightly lighted screen to the total darkness of the room overworks the muscles of the eye pupils and results in fatigue. There is no objection to the use of a filter before the screen, but you should not wear dark glasses while looking at television because they strain your eyes when you turn away to see something in the less brightly lighted sections of the room. Dr. Rones recommends the P4 type of screen, which produces a minimum of eye fatigue and is also well balanced to eliminate "flicker."

KEEP YOUR SET IN FOCUS

Parents with youngsters who sit glued to the television set night after night have inquired how long it is safe to look at television. This depends partly on the individual, says Dr. Rones. Just as some people can take long, brisk walks without getting tired, so some people can give their closest attention to a television program without eye fatigue. It is always wise, however, to rest one's eyes by turning away from the screen at short intervals. (This is, we suggest, perhaps the best excuse for commercials.) Of course it goes without saying that the television set should be kept in the best of condition at all times, so that the focus is always adjusted to the finest possible degree.

Finally, Dr. Rones suggests an aspect of television that had never before occurred to us. Perhaps, he says, it may be a blessing in disguise, for it demands more efficient and accurate use of one's eyes. So if you find that your eyes become easily fatigued by television, it may be a warning that they are not functioning at their best and you should have them tested for minor errors in focus.

SIT ABOUT TEN FEET AWAY

A query on the subject of possible eyesight harm from television is answered in the February 3, 1952, *Journal of the American Medical Association.* The authority who answers the question states that in general, sitting at a distance of 10 feet or more from the screen is best and that you should never sit as close as 5 feet. A distance of roughly 10 times the diameter of the screen is most comfortable for easy viewing and avoidance of eye strain. The *Journal* also suggests that changing from one chair to another from time to time is helpful because it rests the eyes as well as the neck muscles.

The whole question of television in relation to eyesight was covered at a recent annual convention of the New York State Optometric Association. Dr. Irving J. Stone outlined the ideal conditions for television viewing thusly: Television should be watched in a room lighted by a shaded 40-watt bulb to the rear of the viewers. A 10-inch screen should be watched from a distance of 8 feet, a 16-inch screen from 14 feet, and a 24-inch screen from at least 20 feet. So don't envy your neighbor his big television screen if his living room is small. His screen may be larger than yours, but his bills from the optometrist may be larger, too!

We have only one further suggestion to make: If you're so enamored of television that you can't tear yourself away, provide yourself with a bowl of sunflower seeds, rather than pretzels or salted peanuts, while you're watching your favorite programs. In case the television is straining your eyes, the sunflower seeds you munch while you watch will be building them up again.

SPOTS BEFORE THE EYES

A question to the editor of the *British Medical Journal* (April 17, 1954) inquires "What are the causes of 'spots before the eyes'? What are their significance and treatment?" The editor answers that spots before the eyes may be an indication of something generally wrong, such as a disorder of the blood vessels or the liver. Or it may be the result simply of opaque spots in the vitreous, or transparent, part of the eye, in which case they are completely harmless and nothing to worry about.

There is a possibility, of course, that they may come from quite serious eye diseases, such as choroidoretinitis (inflammation of the retina) or a detached retina. In these cases they do not generally seem to be just plain "spots" but shimmering lights, halos around things at night, and other manifestations of something wrong with the eyes.

The editor tells us that there is no treatment for spots before the eyes. First, of course, one should have an eye examination. If nothing is amiss with the eyes, a general examination should reveal whether there is a disorder of the blood vessels, the liver, and so forth. If all the tests are negative, then it seems best to ignore the spots because they do not signify anything important, says the editor.

A friend of ours who had vivid flashing spots of light before her eyes went to an oculist; he could find nothing wrong with her eyes, and he said goodby to her in these words, "If you find out what causes it, let me know. I've had just such spots for the past five years." A general examination showed that she had an abscessed tooth which had spread infection throughout her body and resulted in anemia, as well as deficiency in all the vitamins and minerals. After the tooth came out, a good diet with supplements of vitamins A, B, C, and D and bone meal dissolved the spots in a few weeks.

Incidentally, when I was a young man I had spots

before my eyes. I went to an oculist who gave me drops which I swallowed in water. In a few days the spots disappeared. This was in 1919. Today old-fashioned medicine is a forgotten art.

EYECUPS

A note in the New Hampshire *Health News* points out that the eyecup is in the same category as the family toothbrush—a menace to health. Dr. Cogwell, author of the article, reminds us that infection of one kind or another can be easily transferred by using a common eyecup, so the gadget should always be boiled or sterilized before using.

But perhaps more important is the fact that there doesn't seem to be much sense in using an eyecup at all—even a sterilized one. The eye secretes a liquid called lysozyme. This enzyme is a powerful antiseptic against most bacteria. Left to itself, it will probably take care of whatever is bothering the eye; why wash it away?

BELLADONNA HARMS EYES

In the *American Journal of Ophthalmology* for May, 1950, Drs. E. V. Ullman and F. D. Mossman tell of treating six patients for serious eye trouble which seemed to be the consequence of the taking of belladonna. All of the patients had been prescribed belladonna by physicians who had been treating them for gastrointestinal disorders that ranged from duodenal and peptic ulcers to colitis and hyperacidity. These patients were also all in the stage of life in which the type of ocular ailment afflicting them occurs, that is, from 38 to 68 years old. The ophthalmologists discovered that they had acquired glaucoma, a dread eye disease in which the eyeball hardens, pressure within it increases, and ultimate blindness ensues. However, since they had not had the opportunity to examine any of the six patients before their own physicians had treated them with belladonna, Drs. Ullman and Mossman cannot state dogmatically that either the drug or an overdose of it had precipitated the glaucoma, though in all cases the first symptoms of ocular disorder had occurred in the patients within a few days or weeks after the administration of the medicament.

The prescribing physicians seem to have been negligent in failing to question their clients on any past history of eye trouble they may have had, though, of course, it is possible that they did not know that belladonna can have this dangerous side effect. Since, however, the ophthalmologists cite figures showing that roughly one-fourth of the cases of glaucoma which they treated were either brought on or intensified by the use of belladonna, and since other eye doctors may for years have been treating victims of the disease without knowing that they were belladonna users, the drug is definitely questionable, if not outright pernicious.

123

Chapter 17

Troubles with the Eyes

It is noteworthy that fatigue and eyestrain are the principal reasons for headaches, according to the people interviewed in a survey we conducted. Some medical opinions agree with this, other doctors disagree. Dr. Francis M. Walsh, of the University of Minnesota, and Dr. Leon D. Harris, of the Lutheran Deaconess Hospital, Minneapolis, writing in *Modern Medicine* for March 1, 1952, say that actual eye disorders are quite infrequent among children brought to them. Studying 100 young patients from four to seventeen years of age, they found that 46 had "depressed" vision but were free from any other symptoms. The remaining 54 had normal vision without glasses but were brought to the doctor complaining of headaches, eyes that hurt, being slow readers, and holding books close to their eyes while reading.

"Children with good vision may complain of headaches, of eye pain, to gain parental attention," say these physicians, and "the first-born whose place is usurped by a new baby . . . may feel neglected and sometimes resorts to this stratagem." In the opinion of these doctors, slow reading and holding books close to the eyes are caused by other things entirely, and they seem to feel that getting glasses for the child will not effect cures. Emotional origin is far more common in such headaches.

On the other hand, Dr. Albert D. Ruedmann, professor of ophthalmology at Wayne University School of Medicine, declared in the October 14, 1952, issue of the *Journal of the American Medical Association* that 25 per cent of all headaches are caused by eye difficulty. He said that eyes are overworked, overused, and used under poor working conditions (bad light, etc.). He gave as examples the child who is inattentive, the businessman who has a headache at noon which is relieved by lunch and then has a recurrence about 3 or 4 o'clock in the afternoon, the convalescent patient who reads in bed, and so forth.

They may require, he said medical exercises, surgical treatment, glasses, or all three. He also believes that pains in the neck which may lead to headache are caused by imbalance in the muscles of the eyes. The neck muscles function chiefly to move the head so that the eyes are in good position to see. If there is a disorder in the balance of the eye muscles, the neck muscles must be strained to get good sight.

BLOODSHOT EYES

A Cincinnati physician writes to the editor of the *Journal of the American Medical Association,* July 24, 1954, commenting on chronic bloodshot eyes. If no weakening chronic disease is present to account for the bleary-looking orbs, he says, it is very possible that the patient has not been getting enough of the right kind of nutrition. Omitting alcohol and putting the patient on a diet high in vitamins, with particular attention to the B vitamins, may correct the condition entirely. So before you decide that your neighbor with the bloodshot eyes probably spends most of his time bending an elbow at the local bar, why not suggest helpfully to his wife that she begin to serve more liver and get into the habit of using brewer's yeast in some way or other in the family's meals. Any good book on nutrition at the local library will tell her what other foods are rich in the B vitamins.

I, too, used to suffer from bloodshot eyes occasionally, but since eating sunflower seeds this no longer occurs.

Chapter 18

What to Do for an Eye Condition

A MAN FROM FLORIDA whom I have known personally and who grows his own vegetables organically
wrote me as follows:

"Last week I returned from Johns Hopkins in Baltimore, where I went to one of the nation's outstanding eye specialists, having developed 'light flashes' in
one of my eyes, I find from his examination that I'm
a candidate for a detached retina. I immediately returned home and secured a vegetable juicer, and am
drinking 'gobs' of carrot and celery juice, and almost
everything else I can lay my hands on.

"While I know you are not a doctor, I am fully
aware you have had quite a range of experience in
various physical disabilities, and am wondering if any
such case as this has come under your study and
observation. Certainly it is very distressing to be con-
fronted with the possibility of an operation, or the

loss of my sight. I will appreciate it if you will give me any suggestions, in the event you are familiar with this sort of thing."

Here is a résumé of the letter I sent him:

I was sorry to hear about your condition. As you state, I am not a physician and do not know much about conditions such as the one you describe or anything that is in the field that might require surgery. I am not against surgery when it is absolutely necessary, but certainly I am against the easy readiness with which such operations are suggested.

You say that you are a candidate for a detached retina, but you do not have the detached retina now. That sounds better and I believe you ought to go all out for every possible means of improving your health by means of dietary methods.

The first thing I can tell is that the use of sunflower seeds is specific for the eyes. Be sure you eat enough of them.

Definitely, if I were you, I would buy bone meal . . . and take it religiously. Bone meal furnishes, in a natural form, minerals that are needed in every part of the body. You should take vitamin A and D perles made from fish liver oil, but be sure it is a brand that is a natural product and not synthetic. I would also take brewer's yeast.

Then you should get some vitamin C tablets made from rose hips, the little berries or fruit of the rose bush, and you should take vitamin E made from vegetable oils. I would also take garlic perles. Garlic is a very wonderful product, and I have a great deal of medical information in conservative medical journals showing that it cleanses the blood and is generally a good thing to take. I am soon going to have articles on garlic.

You ought to find a source of organically produced meat. Surely somebody in Florida is raising cattle by the organic method. I will make a note to look this up in my records and will write you within a day or so.

Follow the articles in *Prevention* magazine so as to take out of your diet all of the foods in which chemicals have been used during their manufacture. This means to disregard practically all of the foods that come out of factories or out of cans. There is still enough food left to have a happy diet. You can eat fruit, but I would suggest that, in the case of such things as apples and pears, you peel them because of the poison-spray residues. You can never tell but that some of these residues of poison sprays may be contributing to your condition. There are plenty of vegetables to be eaten and I am very much in favor of meat and, of course, fruits.

In your case I think it is very important that your eyes are not subject to cigarette or cigar smoke. Many people today, I am sure, get trouble in their eyes due to the terribly irritating effect of tobacco smoke. I don't know whether you are a smoker personally—if you are, you ought to give it up. Many people also have their eyes irritated by tobacco smoke by going

129

to certain places of meeting, such as lodges and other places where heavy smoking is going on. Some people play cards where there is much smoking, and this is extremely irritating to the eyes. I think, in your case, you should pay particular attention to this possibility.

I think, also, that it is important that you go on a diet which contains no white sugar and very little of any other sugars, such as honey or blackstrap molasses. The sugar that you need you can get from fruits and the sweeter vegetables. In fact, most of the carbohydrates that you eat turn into sugar. This means cutting out ice cream, pie, cake, soft drinks, and all that sort of stuff. I remember when I had lunch with you that you ordered pie. You rascal!

You should also go on practically a salt-free diet. Salt-free diets are not advisable in some few cases where there are certain diseases. These are very serious diseases and I am sure you do not have them. But in the average case, it is very important ordinarily that both sugar and salt are cut out because they play havoc with your tissues and their functioning. Your eyes have delicate tissues and I can see that it is very important that you cut out salt and sugar, especially in the face of a possible eye involvement.

If you will do all of the things that this letter advises, I feel certain that you will attain a much better bodily health, and it may contribute toward the condition that will prevent your eye trouble from going any further.

You will be amazed how you will gradually get

used to new habits of eating. At first, I had trouble in cutting out such things as ice cream and pies, but now I would rarely think of breaking my training on the score of sweets.

Sincerely yours,
J. I. Rodale

P.S.: Do a lot of walking outdoors.

Here is a letter I sent to my friend on March 25, 1952, a few months after my first letter:

When I returned here I found the following among my papers, and I thought you would be interested. It shows the importance of vitamins in your condition.

FUNDUS OCULI

(From *International Review of Vitamin Research*, Vol. XXIII, No. 1, 1951, page 77), translated from German; an article by E. Heinsius, "The Participation of Nutritional Deficiency in Cases of Fundus Oculi," Allg. Krkhs. Hamburg-Heindberg. Dtsch. md. Wschr 1950.

"A description is given of retina modification, that plays a considerable part in the special aspects of diseases due to nutrition deficiency. It deals with optic nerve modification (loss of color, atrophy, papillary-oedema) and retina damage (maculated retinitis and finally angiospastic retinitis). Vitamin A defi-

131

ciency and disturbance in assimilation of vitamin B is declared responsible for fundus oculi as well as is albumen-loss, hormone disturbance, and environmental influence."

I am convinced that the intensity of the Florida sun has something to do with your condition, and I feel that you ought to protect yourself from the sun as much as possible. I do not think that colored lenses are sufficient because I think the sun penetrates at the side of your face. My suggestion would be to spend as little time as possible outdoors during the time of day when the sun's rays are intense. If you have to work in your garden sometime, wait for twilight. I think you ought to give serious consideration to this angle, and possibly arrange to spend long periods of time up North, if you could so arrange your affairs.

I enjoyed my visit with you and hope to see you again next year, and that your eyes will be in much better shape then.

Best wishes.

Sincerely yours,
J. I. Rodale

Here is his reply:

Dear Friend Rodale:
Well, I'm getting along pretty good. Item number

one is, I haven't had a smoke now in almost three weeks, believe it or not, and that's been a little tough, Brother Rodale, after having puffed on cigars and a pipe for almost fifty years—that's pretty tough. However, I've got that pretty much behind me now, and it's quite possible this will have some beneficial results. Then, in addition to that, I go out here once a week and take a steam bath and a good massage; then I've been running over here to an osteopath, on the assumption his treatment might help my circulation. I've cut down on starches and sweets. I have, as a matter of fact, almost entirely eliminated these very tasty items from my diet, and that too has been a little distressing, because those are the very things I like best. However, they have been just about eliminated. I eat about one slice of whole wheat bread a day, which isn't going in for bread very strong, you'll have to admit.

I imagine all this pretty much conforms to your ideas. I'm eating salads, Brother Rodale, and I mean salads—twice a day, for lunch and for dinner—salads. I got up early this morning and prepared breakfast, and made an omelette, and this omelette would have knocked your eye out. It was made from six eggs from hens which are organically fed, and they even have for dessert some of my ten and fourteen inch earthworms. Now you can imagine what that does to an egg. They are so full of vitamins, vim and vigor that they actually hop up and down when I break them into the frying pan.

Hope this finds you in good health and spirits, and

133

that you have eliminated coffee from your diet.
With kindest personal regards, I remain,

Sincerely yours,

I wrote to my friend about 6 years later and he replied as follows:

Dear Mr. Rodale:

Many thanks for your letter. About my eyes, I went to Dr. Dunnington, at the Presbyterian Hospital, in New York and have returned each year for examination. I have had no further trouble—thank God. I did this, however, I quit smoking five years ago. Thank God for that, also Dr. Dunnington wished me to "cut down" on my smoking. So, I cut it out. I was a heavy smoker—big black cigars. I now have no desire to smoke.

Glad all is well with you. Best Wishes, to you and the family.

Chapter 19

Conclusion

THE MOST IMPORTANT thing I can tell you about the conservation of your eyesight is to watch your nutrition as described in this book, and be sure to eat enough sunflower seeds every day. They should be a substitute for candy and other sweets. Parrots live to ages over 80, happy in the confines of a cage, with little more than sunflower seeds for food.

You will find unexpected dividends if you add this seed to your diet.

Remember that healthy eyes are tied in with a healthy body, so that anything you can do to improve that health will be helpful in maintaining the well-being of your eyes.

Another thing—it may be difficult to adopt a new habit, but if you persevere for a few days you will find it becoming second nature.

As Aristotle said, "That which has become habitual becomes, as it were, natural. In fact, habit is something like nature, for the distance between 'often' and 'always' is not great, and nature belongs to the idea of 'always,' habit that of 'often.' "

If you wish to keep up with my health writings, subscribe to *Prevention*, Emmaus, Pennsylvania. Write for a sample copy.

Index